# Healing in High Gear: Surviving Sepsis, a Guide for Patient Safety, Healing & Advocacy

# Healing in High Gear: Surviving Sepsis, a Guide for Patient Safety, Healing & Advocacy

**AN INSPIRING TRUE STORY OF THE SEPSIS JOURNEY OF JIM HOWELL AND HIS FAMILY**

"Compelling, Terrifying, Helpful...Every patient needs to read this"--Norman
"Every Hospital, Nurse, Doctor, Healthcare worker needs to read this book"--Cindy, RN
"I could not put this book down--I'm buying it for my sister"--Joan
"Life saving information and great resource for all caregivers"--Laura, RN

Foreword by Gary Shorb, CEO Methodist Le Bonheur Healthcare

## Amy Donaho Howell

Portion of Proceeds from each book sale donated to patient advocacy and sepsis awareness

ISBN: 1534960341
ISBN 13: 9781534960343
Library of Congress Control Number: 2016911728
CreateSpace Independent Publishing Platform
North Charleston, South Carolina

S ummary: This book is intended to be an inspirational, truthful and helpful guide to **how to survive** a surgery gone horribly wrong--physically,
mentally, spiritually and financially. This true story will make you believe
in miracles, cry, laugh, strengthen your faith and realize that sometimes--when
you trust your instincts and use your brain--you are both lucky and smart.
This is the story of Jim Howell, 62, who walked into a hospital healthy and
fit (for a "routine preventative surgery") and then spent over 90 days in it undergoing 4 additional surgeries, multiple times in ICU, on a ventilator twice,
dodging death at least 3 times. This is also a story about me, his wife, who
had to put career and business, family all on "pause" to care for him, lead the
charge for removing the first surgeon, and find the team that would work hard
to save him.

The names in this book are real and there is only one fictional name and
that is the name of the first surgeon who we believe was both incompetent
and negligent. This book is not about him, except to say that incompetency
cannot be swept under the rug, ignored or tolerated. PERIOD. Hospitals and
surgery centers simply cannot allow mediocre, unresponsive, or negligent surgeons to operate in their facilities. It is dangerous enough to be operated on by
any surgeon.  Even worse, is if that surgeon is arrogant and will not listen to
the patient's family post-operatively. Confidence is a positive trait. Arrogance
is something that can limit a surgeon's ability to work with a team which can
potentially threaten safety issues. In today's competitive world where information abounds and transparency is king, there is no reason for surgeons to be

arrogant or view their role as "above" everyone else. Yes, they are often the lead on the medical team but that doesn't omit them from a team approach to patient care. If I were a hospital CEO or medical director, I would require team training and communication skills for surgeons including transparent practices, patient relations and family communications.

This book is about what was done post-operatively and how the Howell family shifted into the ultimate "high gear" to save Jim's life and focus on getting through an unimaginable nightmare. This book is written for people out there everywhere who have had a bad experience and need help getting through it. It is also for anyone who is facing any type of invasive surgery as it can be a teaching tool to ensure the best possible outcome for a recovery. This book is meant to encourage and support family members who have questions but are afraid to challenge a doctor to ask them. Expressed in this book are my opinions, observations and conclusions drawn by my personal experience. I have no formal medical training or background other than personal experiences and my professional consulting work with physician practices over the past 20 years.

This book is dedicated to all of the prayer warriors we had (and still have), the medical team that saved Jim, the hospital we love and all of the patient advocates and caregivers who work tirelessly everyday in one of the hardest jobs ever.

# Foreword: By Gary Shorb, CEO, Methodist Le Bonheur Healthcare

Amy Howell's poignant book is about an experience that no individual or family should ever have to endure. For Amy and her husband Jim, their experience with the healthcare system challenged every aspect of their very lives. The good news is that they survived, and now Amy is able to offer insights and advice to benefit others who may face a similar challenge. Unfortunately, those others will number in the hundreds of thousands every year.

I've spent most of my career in the healthcare industry, and over the years, I've repeatedly been struck by the talent and dedication I've seen in healthcare workers, from those who clean and supply hospital rooms to those performing highly specialized surgical procedures. Somehow despite the abilities and commitment of those called to healthcare careers, medical errors in hospitals and health systems are all too common. Just this year, the number one hospital in the country at Johns Hopkins University led a study that showed medical errors in hospitals and health systems may be the third leading cause of death in the United States – claiming 251,000 lives each year, ahead of respiratory disease, accidents, stroke and Alzheimer's. Add to this patient injuries resulting from medical error and the numbers increase as much as forty times.

One of the biggest threats to life is sepsis which is a complication of an infection. It occurs when chemicals released into the bloodstream to fight infection lead to inflammatory responses throughout the body. This inflammation can trigger a cascade of changes that damage multiple organ systems, causing them to fail. This is what happened to Jim, and it nearly killed him. It is extremely important to detect sepsis early as risk of death goes from 30% at its beginning stages to 80% when a patient goes into septic shock. It was Amy's observation of her husband's condition and the medical team's immediate action that saved Jim's life.

That is why this book is so important. Those of us in leadership positions in healthcare know that we must be more aggressive in working to improve patient safety, reduce clinical treatment variability, enhance communication, increase transparency and improve systems of care. Perhaps most importantly, we must do a better job of listening to patients and their families. Progress is being made, but the pace must be accelerated. In the meantime, patients and family members must be advocates for appropriate and safe care. Amy, knowing her husband better than any provider could, intervened on numerous occasions to insure her husband had what he needed when he needed it. Her lessons learned from this experience are insightful and provide extremely valuable and potentially lifesaving advice for anyone dealing with chronic or severe illness. The healthcare industry is committed to doing better, and Amy's experience motivates all of us to accelerate our progress. Books like this offer guidance as to what we need to focus on as providers, family members and patients to transform the industry and ensure the best possible care for patients and their families.

Foreword: By Gary Shorb, CEO, Methodist Le Bonheur
Healthcare · · · · · · · · · · · · · · · · · · · · · · · · · · · · · · · · · · · · · · ix

Chapter Outline:

Preface · · · · · · · · · · · · · · · · · · · · · · · · · · · · · · · · · · · · · · · · · xiii

Chapter 1   The story of Jim Howell: From a "routine" surgery
to hell and back --several times--to tell about it · · · · · · · · · · · · 1

Chapter 2   Sepsis: The Masked Murderer · · · · · · · · · · · · · · · · · · · · · · · 31

Chapter 3   When Tragedy Strikes: Shifting into High Gear Action · · · · · 38

Chapter 4   Stress on the Caregivers:
Support systems, Friends and Coping Tools · · · · · · · · · · · · · 46

Chapter 5   Financial Matters · · · · · · · · · · · · · · · · · · · · · · · · · · · · · · · 55

Chapter 6   Dealing with Hospitals, Medical Teams, Surgeons · · · · · · · · 59

Chapter 7   A word--or several--about Insurance Companies · · · · · · · · · · 68

Chapter 8   How to Survive 90+ days in a Hospital · · · · · · · · · · · · · · · · 72

Chapter 9    Balancing running a Business and your Family
while your Spouse is in the Hospital · · · · · · · · · · · · · · · · · 76

Chapter 10 Hospitals: Transparency and Accountability· · · · · · · · · · · · · 79

Chapter 11 Purpose of this book and How Helping Others Helps You · · 82

Chapter 12 Healing Scripture Verses · · · · · · · · · · · · · · · · · · · · · · · · 84

Chapter 13 The Final Surgery: June 14, 2016 · · · · · · · · · · · · · · · · · · 92

Acknowledgements · · · · · · · · · · · · · · · · · · · · · · · · · · · 95

About the Methodist Foundation · · · · · · · · · · · · · · · · · · · 99

About the author: · · · · · · · · · · · · · · · · · · · · · · · · · · · 101

# Preface

There is so much information online about medical errors, surgical errors and it is apparent to me that we still have a long way to go. The following article is one of the best I found from Leapfrog, an independent, national nonprofit organization advocating for patient safety.

## Hospital Errors are the Third Leading Cause of Death in U.S., and New Hospital Safety Scores Show Improvements Are Too Slow

**Washington, D.C., October 23, 2013** – New research estimates up to 440,000 Americans are dying annually from preventable hospital errors. This puts medical errors as the third leading cause of death in the United States, underscoring the need for patients to protect themselves and their families from harm, and for hospitals to make patient safety a priority.

Released in the Fall of the 2013 update to The Leapfrog Group (Leapfrog) Hospital Safety Score assigns A, B, C, D and F grades to more than 2,500 U.S. general hospitals. It shows many hospitals are making headway in addressing errors, accidents, injuries and infections that kill or hurt patients, but overall progress is slow. The Hospital Safety Score is calculated under the guidance of the Leapfrog Blue Ribbon Expert Panel, with a fully transparent methodology analyzed in the peer-reviewed *Journal of Patient Safety.*

Leapfrog, an independent, national nonprofit organization that administers the Score, is an advocate for patient safety nationwide. "We are burying a population the size of Miami every year from medical errors that can be prevented. A number of hospitals have improved by one or even two grades, indicating hospitals are taking steps toward safer practices, but these efforts aren't enough," says Leah Binder, president and CEO of Leapfrog. "During this time of rapid health care transformation, it's vital that we work together to arm patients with the information they need and tell doctors and hospitals that the time for change is now."

As result of the push for more public reporting of hospitals' safety efforts, Leapfrog added two new measures to the latest Hospital Safety Score release, including Catheter-Associated Urinary Tract Infections (CAUTIs) and Surgical Site Infections: Colon (SSI: Colon). While CAUTIs and SSI: Colon have not received as much public attention as other measures, they are among the most common hospital infections and claim a combined 18,000 lives each year. With data from the CMS Hospital Compare website as well as the Leapfrog Hospital Survey, Leapfrog now has the publicly available data needed to calculate these critical measures into the Score.

CAUTI and SSI: Colon are among the 28 measures of publicly available hospital safety data used to produce a single grade representing a hospital's overall safety rating.

The Hospital Safety Score is a public service available at no cost online. A full analysis of the data and methodology used is also available on the Hospital Safety Score website.

## Key Findings

- On average, there was no improvement in hospitals' reported performance on the measures included in the score, with the exception of hospital adoption of computerized physician order entry (CPOE). The expansion in adoption of this lifesaving technology suggests that federal policy efforts to improve hospital technology have shown some success.

- Of the 2,539 general hospitals issued a Hospital Safety Score, 813 earned an "A," 661 earned a "B," 893 earned a "C," 150 earned a "D" and 22 earned an "F."

- While overall hospitals report little improvement in safety, some individual hospitals (3.5 percent) showed dramatic improvements of two or more grade levels.

- The states with the smallest percentage of "A" hospitals include New Hampshire, Arkansas, Nebraska and New Mexico. No hospitals in New Mexico or the District of Columbia received an "A" grade.

- Maine claimed the number-one spot for the state with the highest percentage of "A" hospitals.

- Kaiser and Sentara were among the hospital systems that achieved straight "A" grades, meaning 100 percent of their hospitals received an "A."

For more information about the Hospital Safety Score or to view the list of state rankings, please visit www.hospitalsafetyscore.org.

The bottom line is that hospitals must balance being efficient and profitable while also being focused on quality patient care. If the goal is to minimize hospital returns and failed outcomes, hospitals must seek better standards in sepsis awareness as well as minimize surgical errors.

# CHAPTER 1

## The story of Jim Howell: From a "routine" surgery to hell and back --several times--to tell about it

> "When you are going through hell...just keep going"
> --WINSTON CHURCHILL

One day you are happy, healthy and vibrant and within a few days you are laying in the ICU with sepsis so bad nobody thinks you will make it. This--in one sentence--is what happened to Jim Howell, age 62, my husband of 22 years and the father of our two children, Bryan (20) Abby (16). I will try and be brief about what happened to us. It is ugly, horrid and something I wouldn't wish on any human--ever.

I kept a daily journal (not because I thought I would need it) but because I am in communications (PR and crisis communications) and I'm also a writer. I'm a natural for writing things down and documenting things. I am not putting the whole journal in this book for many reasons, but I have it. And I will insert little slices of stories from it to illustrate some of the points I want to share in this journey (which is still going as I write this).

What happened? Jim Howell went in for his annual colonoscopy after having some repeat bouts of diverticulitis (a painful infection in the colon often common in aging men) and his GI (gastrointestinal) doctor told us he had a narrow part of his colon which was getting infected, and that a surgeon could cut it out and reattach it and that is was a fairly routine (no surgery should be referred to as routine). He would be in the hospital for a few days and then recovered after a few weeks. The GI doctor recommended a surgeon "Dr. X" and said he did these often and would be a good one to use (note: this is because most physicians are employed by hospital systems and they "self-refer" or "refer within the network" for profit reasons--I think patients should have more choices but this is an entirely different subject). Jim asked a few contacts he knew about this Dr. X and he seemed to check out as a good surgeon (Later, we would believe otherwise). Fast forward to a surgery date set for January 21, 2015.

Thinking Jim would be "out of commission" for a few weeks, we spent the last few nights before surgery having a family dinner with my parents and our children and went to see "American Sniper." We also drove around downtown Memphis on my golf cart and had a fun dinner at one of our favorite spots. It did not occur to me at this point that this would be the last "normal" in our lives for a very long time. Nor did it occur to me that Jim would be so septic in a matter of days that his chances of survival were slim to none. You know when you hear the term "life is short" or "one day you are here, the next you are gone,"--I get that now.

**Excerpts from my journal:** The following pages are excerpts pulled out of my journal as I wrote them. They haven't been edited and I want them here as original posts, so apologies for inconsistencies, abbreviations, etc. The one thing I did do here is omit all of the clinical and medical information that I recorded because it's not relevant and it would be too boring and make this book too long. Suffice it is to say, Jim was on a ton of medications for the many complications he endured.

### January 21, 2015
"*We arrived at Methodist Hospital in Germantown as instructed at 5:00 a.m. to get Jim ready for surgery. After a few hours of what seemed like nine million questions and too much paperwork, he was finally ready to be wheeled into surgery. At approximately 7:50 a.m. I was told in waiting that surgery was underway. Every hour the wait desk would page me to give me the same update that Jim was "still in surgery" and that was all I*

*would get. By 11:30 I was getting nervous--and deep down, this was really my first internally instinctive "red flag" and I called my sister, Heather and one of my good friends, who came to wait with me and brought me food. Finally at almost 1:00 the desk told me Jim was out of surgery and now going to "recovery." Looking back, a great surgeon would have raced out to see the family after such a long surgery. And it was originally explained it would only take a few hours. It took 5! It took 1 HOUR for the surgeon to come talk to me and explain how it went. He told me the surgery went well, he cut about 18" out of his colon and reattached it. Jim was in recovery until around 5:00 p.m. and was then moved up to 4-West (the post-op floor we would later call home). Ironically, Dr. Susan Murrmann--an OB-GYN and surgeon--and more importantly, long time friend had seen me and wanted to know how she could help (Susan would play a pivotal role later).*

*Jim was rolled into room 430 on 4-West and I stayed the night and things seemed to go as they should. Dr. X came by the next day and told Jim another surgeon would be 'taking call' as it was Friday and he would be "off" for the weekend (What an understatement that was!).*

*Friday afternoon, Jim started showing signs of distress. His blood pressure went up, he was terribly swollen around his abdomen (normal given his surgery) and by the afternoon, cardiology was called in to make sure Jim was not having heart problems. A Nurse Practitioner from Stern Cardiovascular was called in, but I had already called Jim's cardiologist, Dr. Dharmesh Patel who was on the phone ordering tests for Jim and trying to rule out blood clots or heart issues. A CT scan was ordered for his chest (but unfortunately not for his abdomen) and long story short, heart problems were ruled out. The medical team filling in for Dr. X said he was just swollen from surgery and was probably having trouble breathing due to excessive amounts of fluid and congestion in his core and around his abdomen. The cardiologist rounding at the hospital ordered Lasix to get some fluid out and Jim was able to get more comfortable. I was worried sick and did not leave his room. The surgeon on call for Dr. X came by and said he'd check in on Saturday and see if Jim would feel like being discharged.*

*Saturday arrived and the surgeon on call did rounds and said Jim looked better and if cardiology agreed, he could be released. Soon, the cardiologist on call came by and agreed, so amazingly, Jim was released from the hospital. We were home by 2:30 in the afternoon after dropping off his prescription for Percocet (for pain).*

*The rest of the day passed with Jim sitting in his chair, taking his pain medicine for the large incision and stitches he had in his abdomen, and he was able to eat soft food and drink gatorade (none of which he should have done, but we didn't know what was happening on the inside).*

*(At some point, Jim's colon either came apart from the site where Dr. X. reattached it or it was never properly attached in that first surgery. So Friday through the weekend, Jim was getting septic and I didn't know it)*

*By Sunday, Jim felt worse, was getting pale but did not have fever--yet. He took a percocet and went to bed only to wake up a few hours later with a fever of 102.7-a giant red flag. I immediately called the after hours number and the "on call" surgeon called back and said that could be a number of things but to give him antibiotics and call first thing the next day.*

*(I realize now that I should have raced him to the ER Sunday night as soon as his fever spiked. Thankfully, I did the next day.) I tried calling Dr. X's office and finally got through to his nurse, explained everything and she said his condition was "normal" and that Dr. X didn't see patients until a 2-week "post-op" appointment which she said she'd schedule. I explained to her Jim needed to be seen and that I was going to bring Jim in. Her response: "Dr. X has things to do and he's not here--he has other procedures." This was the 14th call that Monday that I had made to Dr. X's trying to get him--and not once did he call me back that morning.*

*What made me think Jim was septic was that I had a friend in the medical field who had warned me that sepsis could happen if the colon wasn't attached or could burst. When I could not get Dr. X to respond, I sent her a text. She immediately called me and said "Get Jim to the Emergency Room Now!" I did exactly that. Our son Bryan (who at the time was in his senior year at Houston High) helped me get him there and wheeled him into the ER.*

*Exactly as we were wheeling a lifeless Jim into the ER (sometime after lunch maybe 1:30) my cell phone rang. It was Dr. X I said, "I am at the ER with Jim and I think he's in serious trouble and I can't talk right now." I hung up and directed all my energy and passion into explaining to ER that I thought Jim was fully septic and that he needed an abdominal CT scan ASAP. His blood pressure was 50/20 if that, and he was now unresponsive, pale and struggling to breathe. I remember that moment vividly. They cut his favorite "Patagonia" shirt off him and went to work. Thankfully I didn't panic or faint. I just calmly told the ER team what I knew and what I thought. One of the nurses asked if I was a doctor. I had a really bad feeling about this and watched while the ER team did their work.*

*The Methodist Le Bonheur Germantown ER doctor probably was one of the first in line to help save Jim. And importantly, she listened to me! I briefed her, she ordered the CT and in what was probably a few hours, but seemed like an eternity, she had the results. Her words to me: "your husband's abdominal cavity is a train wreck and he is fully septic. We will do what we can." If you Google "mortality rate for sepsis" you will see that Jim's chances to live were slim to none.*

*(From here, things happened so fast--and the story is really just beginning so I am going to list out in short order a timeline and what happened over the next days and what turned into a long hospital stay)*

*Monday in ER: Jim was put on all kinds of machines and IVs with the ER team trying to stabilize him. At 8:30 PM Jim was moved to ICU. Around 11:00 PM the nurse on duty (Ben) said he was putting a call into Dr. X to see if he could give Jim more fluid as his pressure remained low all night. The alerts went off 8-10 times and his blood pressure (BP) hovered at 90/60--sometimes lower. Dr. X never called ICU and I know this because I was there and asked Ben specifically if he had called back. Each time, Ben said, "no, he hasn't called us back." ICU's challenge: balancing pain medication with fluids and BP. Jim was in terrible pain and I was completely helpless and alone. I spent the night with Jim in ICU in a chair with my laptop and my brain on high alert--mapping out a strategy of action to save him.*

*Tuesday, Jan. 27: I called in all of Jim's regular M.D.s (Dr. Marty Weiss, internal medicine; Dr. Dharmesh Patel, cardiology; and Susan Murrmann, OB-GYN and friend). Drs. Weiss and Murrmann had called in infectious disease and blood expert, Dr. Threlkeld and also Dr. Sanjeev Mittal, nephrologist. Jim's kidneys were shutting down and by Tuesday morning he was dehydrated. Dr. Mittal ordered a dialysis catheter put in Jim's neck for emergency dialysis. Dr. X was treating Jim with drains and had no sense of urgency nor did he have plans for emergency surgery that Jim desperately needed.*

*Wednesday, Jan. 28: Jim's kidneys shut down and dialysis started. The CEO of the hospital sent me an answer to my email and sent their Chief Medical Director, Dr. Paul Douthitt down to see me. My email was a request to change surgeons immediately, remove Dr. X from the case completely. I signed paperwork and met the Chief of ICU, Dr. Ellis who reversed Dr. X's "step down" orders. Thanks largely to Dr. Murrmann and the hospital administration, we secured Dr. Mark Miller as our new surgeon and I had the attention and support of the hospital administration--a critical key to advocacy.*

*Methodist moved at light speed and by 2:00 Wednesday, Dr. X was being removed from the case and Dr. Miller was on his way to see me. Meanwhile Jim was getting blood, dialysis was starting and Jim's status was in decline. We were in a fast race to save Jim, and Dr. Miller knew it.*

*I liked Dr. Miller at first sight and I will never forget meeting him. He came walking up wearing cowboy boots and scrubs, shook my hand, gave me a smile and said, "I am a straight shooter and I like to tell my patients the truth. Jim's in bad shape. He won't make it if I don't do surgery in the next 24 hours. We have to get him stable enough, his kidneys have shut down, and I have to clean out the sepsis. The surgery could likely kill Jim,*

*but not having it most certainly will kill him," said Miller. I said, "OK,
let's do it." Dr. Miller told me to hang in there and get ready. I could not
believe what was happening but it was happening.*

*Thursday, Jan. 29: SURGERY DAY! I arrived at 8:00 in ICU to find
Dr. Mittal starting another dialysis that would get Jim stable enough for
surgery. All of our friends were gathered in ICU waiting, and looking
back, the support from friends is one of the things that carried me through.
At 1:00 Dr. Miller came and told me he had to take Jim back right now
or he would not make it. I said a prayer and Jim was taken to surgery
which lasted 2 hours--it felt like an eternity.*

*4:00: Dr. Miller came to report (to the whole waiting room of friends and
family) that he got most of the sepsis out, Jim's abdominal cavity was in
bad shape, he had to put drains in and that his colon had come apart at
some point and said it was just raining sepsis in his abdominal cavity. He
compared it to a busted pipe in our house, raining water all over. Jim was
on a ventilator in ICU looking like death and Dr. Miller said the next 48
hours would tell the story and were critical. His words were "I did what I
could, I cleaned him out and had to do a colostomy and we'll worry about
the colon later--might have to go in again...but for now he needs to heal,
he's critical and we don't need any complications. Every hour is critical."*

*At this point, it was starting to sink in that we were in deep trouble and
on a different path than we had planned. Our children were holding up
and our friends and family had surrounded us--helping, sitting in waiting with us, getting my kids food gift cards and gas cards so they could
get food and get to school. I had arranged for Abby to be picked up from
home to get to school and our whole family was now living through an
unimaginable nightmare. The doctors were all there daily checking on
Jim and me and I believed Jim now had a chance. If he could fight, this
team could help him. I am glad I am writing a journal because the days
are running together.*

*Jan. 30-31: Jim made it the critical 48 hours on a ventilator and sedated
in ICU. Dialysis was set for every other day and as needed. He was*

hooked up to so many things it was almost impossible to fathom. He had an open abdominal wound with a "wound vac" attached to help pull fluid and heal. The wound was sort of shaped like an eggplant if that gives you a picture of size. It had to be cleaned and changed by the Methodist wound care team about 3 times a week. He also had an ostomy bag to the left of the wound which also needed cleaning and emptying often. He was on all kinds of IV antibiotics and fluids and had drains literally coming out of him for sepsis.

These 2 days were filled with friends at the hospital bringing food and sitting with me. I managed to get home most nights late because there was really no place to sleep in ICU and I had my kids at home to think about. I kept thinking how grateful I was that Bryan was old enough to drive and his common sense and help through the whole ordeal was incredible.

Sunday, Feb. 1: I could not believe it is Super Bowl Sunday. Dr. Miller told me that today is the first day he believes Jim is "out of the woods" and showing signs of progress. "Baby steps" as he said to me countless times. At 3:15 ICU was able to get Jim off the ventilator. A whole room of friends in the waiting area let out a cheer of joy! Jim could breathe on his own.

The nurse came to get me and when I saw Jim laying there, I said "Honey, hey, it's so great to see you and I love you." Jim looked at me and said in a whisper "Kill me…kill me," I said, "What? Oh no honey somebody already tried that and it didn't work. You are going to be fine. This is just temporary." I guess when you don't really remember what happened and you can't understand what is happening you assume the worst. I think Jim woke to think he was in some type of permanent vegetative state. Jim was in terrible pain, very weak and could hardly swallow but got some water down. When Bryan and Abby came in to see Jim, we all cried tears of joy when Jim responded, "I love you too, more than you can imagine." WOOO HOOO!

I was with lots of friends and family in ICU waiting room for the 1st half of the Super Bowl, and eventually got home to my own bed happy for Jim's progress and praying hard for our family and the medical team.

*I remember specifically praying for God to help me with medical decisions and what we should do in case of the worst. Jim did have a living will and I can't tell you how important it is to understand someone's wishes before they cannot express them for themselves. Jim had told me in the past that he wanted a DNR order (do not resuscitate) should he be in some permanent or prolonged state of ventilator or vegetated. All of these things haunt me daily.*

*Feb. 2: Dropped Abby at school at 7:45 and drove straight to ICU which became my daily routine so I wouldn't miss rounds where the doctors came by to update us. Dr. Mittal was starting dialysis again as Jim's kidneys were still shut down. "Jim's kidneys are strong and they will wake up and everything will be fine. It could be a week, a month or 6 months but everything will be fine," said Dr. Mittal--a very compassionate and wonderful man we grew to love. Dr. Miller seemed pleased and said drains were working and there were likely still "pockets of sepsis" but he would watch it and treat as needed.*

*Feb. 3: A good day! Set my alarm for 5:45 to wake Bryan. The kids were exhausted but hanging tough. Determined to stay "up" for them, I got everyone off to school and arrived at ICU at 8:00 to see Jim sitting up in bed, eyes open and alert. I put my stuff down, walked over to him and said "good morning!" He looked at me and said, "what the hell happened?" This was music to my ears! A flood of emotions took over and I felt like I would faint so I sat down in the chair and thought--for the first time--we will make it through this. Dr. Weiss came in and said he was pleased with Jim's progress and his numbers looked better. Dr. Miller came in and said to Jim, "brother, you made it off death's door several times and I'm happy to say you are going to live and totally recover."*

*Physical therapy came and Jim got out of the bed for the first time in weeks to get to a chair. I can't believe how weak Jim has become only after a few weeks. Baby steps.*

*Feb. 4-6: Dialysis continued, Jim's main issues were kidneys, hydration, PT, strength and no complications. Dr. Mittal ordered dialysis every other day and 30-40 oz of fluid daily to flush kidneys. "I want to see pee," said Dr. Mittal.*

*Feb. 5: We must have been back on 4-West and out of ICU because my diary reports that I was sleeping on the cot in Jim's room helping him get up to pee at night and making sure he didn't fall over his wound vac cords, etc. About 8:00 a.m. Dr. Miller came in to give us the forecast: Jim would be in the hospital for at least 10 more days until he's stronger, followed by months of recovery at home with the colostomy bag and then later--maybe 6-12 months--Dr. Miller would go back in and reverse the colostomy and fix everything and sew him back up. Jim is able to eat a soft GI diet and is feeling better.*

*Feb.7: Jim had to have fluid drained off his lung--a lot of it in CT and also a dialysis treatment. So Jim was gone from his room most of the day and finally returned around 6:00 p.m. He was also given blood and things seemed to look good.*

*Feb. 8: ABBY turned 15!! Woke up to a text from Jim's sister, Julia who had taken a shift to spend the night so I could get a break and it was Abby's birthday. Jim had to have xanex and was anxious, fidgety and uncomfortable. Dr. Miller came by and said they needed to drain a hematoma and Julia stayed. Abby was having her birthday party at Mona Spa where she and 3 friends got masks, eyebrow wax and pampering--thanks to Mona! The spa outing was then followed by a friends and family (including my parents) lunch at a local mexican place of Abby's choosing. In spite of Jim being so ill, I was determined to give Abby a great birthday.*

*Later in the day, I got to the hospital to find that they had drained his hematoma, given him Dilaudid for pain he was in. Dr. Patel was there alarmed to see Jim's hematocrit blood numbers which were not coming up as they should after getting blood. Dr. Patel told me his concern about Jim's blood (DIC), infection and his kidneys. He suggested I stay with Jim at all times to watch him close and help the nurses where I could. It takes a team and more about that later.*

*I was sitting by myself in Jim's room when Dr. Weiss called my cell. Both he and Dr. Miller thought Jim had suddenly worsened and wanted him back in ICU.*

*Our preacher, Will Jones from GPC happened to come in at that time and prayed with me for whatever God wants. Tears streamed down my face and I just could not stop crying--flood gates had opened. I called the kids who came up to see Jim before he went back to ICU. Jim smiled best he could but didn't seem to know it was Abby's birthday. When they left, Abby said, "Mom, it's going to be ok. It's in God's hands," as she hugged me I thought "how am I blessed with such great kids?" I hung onto Abby's sweet faith that day, her birthday. Amazing lessons of faith.*

*By this time, we had a texting strategy and so people knew Jim was headed back to ICU. As they were moving Jim to ICU, friends started popping by like great jolts of energy for me. Sammie McClanahan always showed up at the right times, selflessly staying with Jim, bringing him food, bringing me food. Such a gift. With Jim going back to ICU, I went home and kept my cell charged, on and by my bed.*

*Feb. 9: Woke up at 4:00 a.m. worried about Jim and never went back to sleep. Bryan got up and left at his usual time for school and I showered and went downtown for a client meeting regarding a big real estate project on tap. I took my intern with me to make sure I didn't miss anything and to take notes. It's also good experience for interns to attend client meetings. When I got back out to ICU Jim was doing dialysis again--twice in twelve hours--to get blood and platelets. Dr. Murrmann had Dr. Mike Jones (hematologist) on the case who is one of the best. Later in the day, one of the ICU nurses (with a bad attitude) failed to answer some questions and later told me that Dr. Ellis was "stepping Jim down and out of ICU." I immediately called Dr. Douthitt, medical director, to voice my concern about springing Jim from ICU and stated we needed some consistency of steady numbers and progress before we just let him go back to a regular room. I enlisted the help of Dr. Weiss who agreed and the team eventually agreed Jim could stay in ICU one more night. The RN then suggested that*

*I "not miss any 8:00 rounds" as that is when information is given out. Infuriating thing to say to me, as this was the first day I had to miss rounds due to work. I was quick to point out to him that I had not missed rounds in 19 consecutive days. (Note: when you are advocating for a patient that is moving around within the hospital, you have new medical staff that may not be familiar with case. Patient advocacy meant I had to be there to be Jim's voice and coordinate calls--like a quarterback).*

*Feb. 10: Raced to get Abby to school and to the hospital so as to not miss rounds. Jim was up and wanting to get into a chair so his ICU RN Debbie and I got him up and into the chair with great difficulty. Dialysis was to continue and Dr. Mittal brought paperwork for the eventual out-patient dialysis we were prepared to do upon leaving the hospital--which I was beginning to think would be never.*

*Feb. 11: Jim moved out of ICU and back to 4-West. I got up early to get Abby to school by 7:00 for a test review session so I was at the hospital by 7:15--shift change. Went up to ICU to find out they had moved Jim at 11:00 p.m. but I didn't know this. Went to 4-West to find Jim in room 427 with one of our many favorite nurses, Kari. Jim was up, drinking coffee and ate some ice cream, a few bites of eggs and hash browns (the RNs of 4 West need their own TV show).*

*PT was hard and he walked the floors with a walker in great pain. Baby steps. He had dialysis again at 2:00 (which will wear you out anyway and it was taking a toll although necessary) and my sister Blythe drove from Columbia, SC to be with me! We went to eat while Jim was in dialysis (2 hours usually). After making sure Jim had oxygen on (he tended to pull if off) and meds were set (we talked to the RNs constantly), we left to get home.*

*An arctic blast was headed our way. The weather was getting colder and snow was predicted, although in Memphis that snow often misses us.*

*Feb. 12: Long day! Dropped Abby at 7:30 and got a call from Jim's nurse that Jim had suffered a setback, was in major pain, had blood in his stool and that they were taking him to CT for an abdominal CT. I reminded her "no contrast in CT" (which hurts kidneys). She confirmed that was correct in the orders. I told her I'd be there asap and I was.*

*Arrived to find Jim back on the "evil drug" Dilaudid (when you need it you need it but it did crazy things to Jim). CT revealed blood in abdomen but it was draining on its own, so Dr. Miller was not as concerned. The main concern was another large amount of fluid in Jim's left lung. CT drained 750 cc's of fluid. Very painful and Jim was back on pain meds. Dr. Miller said, "Up, down, up, down...we need more periods of stable." I asked Dr. Miller if I should do an Indian Dance or set up a bar in the shower....joking, he said it wouldn't be a bad idea and that he'd stock it. Laughing, we prayed hard for Jim.*

*Feb. 13: Cold air blast arrived and Abby was out of school. Bryan slept in so I let him miss school. They would also be out Monday for President's Day so it would be a good 4-day stint of sleeping and recovery. I arrived at hospital at 8:30 with Chick-Fil-A for the nurses and they had just taken Jim down for a 3 hour dialysis. So my sister Blythe came up and we went to Hobby Lobby to get Valentines Day decorations for Jim's room and some colored lights. We had also did set up a bar in the bathroom (we didn't really use it much--a few times) and decided if we have to be IN the hospital, we might as well make it as cheery as possible. I had mentioned to Lacey Washburn and Sarah Womack that we "needed a bar in the shower." It wasn't long before Lacey brought the goods. It was happy times and I knew we wouldn't really use it, but it was there as "normal." We need normal. The kids had made some posters for his room with funny sayings on them and scripture to remind Jim of their love and support.*

*Later, the bar would be a big hit by some of the friends we had in and some of the other patient's families. We found people on our floor we knew and the bar was a welcome sight to some of their adult relatives. Although no real amounts of alcohol were consumed there, it was uplifting to know it was there and comical if nothing else. Soon the RN's and medical staff heard about it and would sneak in to take a peek of the bar. I think we had a few bloody mary's from time to time but that was it. All I can say is that it was something sort of fun and it looked cool.*

*That night I spent the night in Jim's room and helped Jim eat, tried to cheer him up. The kids came by but Jim wasn't in a good mood and so they left. Dilaudid helped Jim rest and we got about 4 hours of sleep.*

*Feb. 14: VALENTINE'S Day! In the hospital! It had become a habit for me to walk the halls in my Ralph Lauren pajamas and cowboy boots in search of bad hospital coffee brewing in the break rooms. I mastered making it and try to help out and make a new pot whenever possible for others. Determined to have a fun day, I found the coffee, poured it in my new YETI and put milk and sweetener in it to disguise the burned coffee taste those commercial machines make. Actually it's not that bad and I found myself feeling grateful to have it.*

*The day was a "fun" day considering. Jim was feeling better, our friends Patti and Mike Clauss dropped by with food, Jim's sister Julia brought chocolate covered strawberries...My friend Leslie Schutt arranged for Valentines cards, gifts and flowers for me and the kids...And finally, we took a selfie for Facebook and sent it to Kemp and Anne Conrad--who were also spending Valentine's Day in the hospital (a different one) with a caption that said, "we should NOT make a habit of valentine selfies in the hospital."*

*Feb. 15: Spent all day with Jim and Dr. Murrmann who came up to chat and we had a great time catching up while Jim slept. Later in the day I was whipped and Jim's sister was coming to relieve me. I headed home to find weather forecast calling for snow to which I exclaim, "LET IT SNOW!" I built a fire in my fireplace at home and watched a movie until I couldn't push sleep out any further. Making sure my cell phone was fully charged and on, I put it in it's normal spot beside the bed and crawled into it.*

*Feb. 16: Woke up to sleet hitting the window at 5:00 am but went back to sleep knowing kids were out for the holiday and I prayed for everyone to sleep late. About 9:00 I finally dragged myself out of bed to find coffee and let 3 dogs out. Poor Jim's sister was stuck at the hospital in some iced in conditions so knowing she was there, I enjoyed a leisurely shower. At noon,*

*Bryan drove me in the ice to the hospital. He's a great driver. Somehow the male gender gets a gene that allows them to instinctively know how to guide 4-wheel vehicles in the ice. Abby had spent the night at a friend's, so there was no pressure to be anywhere or get anyone anywhere. I spent the day at the hospital with Jim who was doing better each day. Seemed we were finally seeing pockets of progress but I was beginning to think this will never end.*

*Snow started and by Monday night the schools had announced no school for the next day. YAY! Abby stayed another night with her friend Somer and I slept soundly in my own bed while snow fell outside. Only it was mostly ice.*

*Tuesday, Feb. 17: Woke early and felt the need to get to the hospital. I stopped to get Jim a smoothie with protein, doing my best not to bust my butt on the ice. When I got to Jim's room, he was up and was issuing orders to PT telling them he didn't like their inconsistent schedule and he wanted to know what time they would be there each day. I took this as a positive sign. He also told them he wanted a sheet of paper that had the important exercises on them so he could do on his own (which he could hardly do). Then he told dietary this: "The food you serve here is crap and you need to quit bringing trays of it to me." This was about the only time Jim got a bit feisty as he was really a fantastic patient.*

*When a patient has so many issues like Jim did, diet and nutrition play a key role. Luckily I was aware of it, doing research and getting good information from some of my friends (Leslie Schutt) and we were bringing Jim very "gut healing" foods. Probiotics, protein smoothies, etc. Paul and Jennifer Chandler loaned me their super "vitamix" and I was studying things to make for Jim.*

*The ice outside--although dangerous--has been a blessing to me. School has been cancelled for the following day!*

*Wed. Feb. 18: More snow fell and woke up around 7:00 to a quiet house and two sleeping teens. Arrived at the hospital around 9:00 with a protein smoothie for Jim to find our friends the Sappenfield's there visiting with Jim. Jim needed a shave badly but with 2 neck "ports" still in him, shaving was not an option.*

*Over the next few days, Jim improved and Dr. Miller said he could go home Saturday, Feb. 21. He would need home care (more on that later) and would leave with a wound vac attached to him, his ostomy and pain meds. It has been a long month!*

*The few days that followed at home were basically good. For me, it was like having a new baby because I had to help Jim up to pee and help carry his wound vac (which has a motor that purrs all night but you get used to it) and basically wait on him. But it truly felt so good to be HOME.*

*One of my duties is to empty Jim's ostomy bag. This is truly testing the "for better for worse" in a marriage. You do what you have to do and this became pretty routine and not too bad actually. Never in my wildest dreams would I think we'd be doing this but there we were! The next few days are a blur but I managed to write in my journal and our days were spent 100% focused on Jim's needs. Home health came and went and trained me on how to do what they were doing. My house went from looking like my home to a clinic filled with boxes, supplies, equipment, etc. You wouldn't believe the all of the medical supplies it takes to help someone like Jim. My sister brought over an electric recliner which was the only thing Jim could be comfortable in.*

*It just kept snowing. Monday, Feb. 23 the kids were out again and I built a fire in the fireplace and got Jim up and in front of it. We talked about what happened and spent the day inside with the kids. This was a critical day. Bryan told Jim he'd changed his mind and instead of going to college at MS State, he would apply to University of Memphis instead--for a lot of reasons. We discussed it and concluded Memphis would be a great choice and, frankly, one we could afford--hopefully.*

*Feb. 24: Home health came and changed out the wound vac and ostomy. Jim seemed very tired and the RN said that for every one day in a hospital, it takes three to recover.*

*6:00 PM: Jim's wound vac stopped working. Thankfully, they had trained me on what to do if that happened. Like magic my friend Bridget walked in my door (with soup and food) and immediately donned surgical gloves to assist me in changing out Jim's wound. When a wound vac "stops" you must remove it from the wound (lots of tape and dressings) and re-pack the wound with sanitized saline and wound dressings and tape it all back up. Bridget and I managed this and about half way through it (you have to laugh or you will cry), Bridget said, "this reminds me of tending to my horses but the only difference is that Jim Howell is not biting and kicking us." Thank God for friends with a sense of humor!*

*I guess now that we were at home, people were bringing food which was a great help as I had two eating machines as teens in my house.*

*Just as things were seeming to settle back down.....it changed overnight.*

*Feb. 25: Jim woke with fever 102. Per Dr. Miller, back to the ER we went! Bryan drove us again. It seemed like it took forever in ER where they tested for sepsis and did another abdominal CT scan and blood cultures. Finally at 1:00 AM we were were admitted to the 3rd floor "step down" where I didn't know any of the RNs and had to spend time bringing them up to speed on what had happened. Over the next few days, Jim stayed on 3 and I was able to give him a bath because the 3rd floor rooms have seats in the shower (Note: all showers should have seats for patients who cannot stand long). I requested a transfer to 4-West where all the RNs knew us and were familiar with Jim's case. Consistency of care is the goal.*

*Feb. 26-March 3: were spent back in the hospital on 4-West with Jim eating, trying to walk (very weak) and treating infection that just won't go away. Finally, we were allowed to go back home and it was raining so hard in front of a massive, approaching snowstorm. We packed Jim in my car--still weak but homebound again.*

*March 4: Snow, snow and more snow! The kids were again out of school and I took care of Jim and cooked. I made chili and mashed potatoes--the ultimate snow and comfort food in our house. Our friend Rob Thompson--who was also a fixture in the hospital--came over and we propped Jim in the sunlight as it eventually streamed across the snow filled backyard into our kitchen. I posted a photo of Jim sitting in the kitchen in that light on my Facebook page and everyone was so happy to see Jim sitting there in the light--at home!*

*March 5: HELL DAY! Before I tell you about what happened to Jim.... here I will insert what actually happened to me. I haven't told many people about this but it happened. I woke up before Jim and laid in the bed beside him listening to the wound vac purr and feeling like Bryan or Abby had crawled in our bed behind me. I thought "why is Bryan in our bed" because I could literally feel a pressure and warmth from my head to my toes and I knew it had to be my tall Bryan. Whoever it was--he or she was longer than me--almost holding me all the way around. I remember not wanting to move, not wanting to disturb such a comfort so I just laid there feeling nothing but pure bliss. It was a real power and I felt it--physically. It felt comforting, warm and all I remember is not wanting it to end. Reluctantly, I rolled over and when I did, it was gone. At first I was afraid. Then, I truly believe God's angel was there embracing me as a sign for what was about to happen......What other explanation could there be? If that is 1/10th of what heaven feels like, I'm all in! (note: I have wanted that angel back many times but haven't had it but I thank God for sending it on this day).*

*Here is what happened next:*

*Jim got up to pee at 6:30 a.m. and as he bent down to pick up the wound vac that he had to carry with him, his blood pressure had dropped, he got dizzy and fell hard in our bedroom. As he landed, he fell into a wood chest and hit the floor so hard that the wound vac box came clean apart. His fall was followed by a scream of pain I have never heard from Jim. Bryan heard it and came bolting downstairs to help me get him up and into bed. Terrible pain ensued and Jim announced he was going into shock. He knew the feeling (from his rugby days) and I took his pressure and it was 80/20. He was clammy and I called 911 this time. Then I called Dr. Miller who said he'd meet us in the ER. Finally an ambulance made it's way into our icey, snowy drive and Bryan helped the EMT's get Jim into the ambulance where they immediately started working on him. I told the EMT's everything I knew about Jim and told them to treat for sepsis and shock.*

*As the ambulance left, I told the kids I needed a shower and needed Bryan to then take me to the ER. Thank goodness we had called the ambulance. Police had closed all the roads around us and we had to backtrack many times to finally get to the hospital. It was the first time I have ever seen the police actually close Houston Levee Road.*

*We got to the ER and my college friend, Tripp was the ER physician on duty. Tripp and I went to Rhodes college together and although I don't see him, I sure was glad to see him on this day. He said, "Amy, Jim's in big trouble--he's bleeding internally and Dr. Miller is looking at this closely." Dr. Miller met me at ER and after tests and conferring with the medical team, we were back in ICU facing critical emergency surgery AGAIN.*

*I could not believe it. This time, Jim was in CV-ICU (Cardiovascular ICU) on the first floor--a different ICU than last time. Here it was a Friday and I sent texts to my support team telling them Jim was in trouble again and where I was. It didn't take long for my friends to show up and at about 2:30 Dr. Miller came to find me. He was in his scrubs and said these words: "We are going to surgery this afternoon or Jim will not live." Immediately Jim was wheeled into surgery where Dr. Miller would open him up--yet again--clean out the blood and try and stop wherever it was coming from. His expression said it all and I just nodded and thought, "how are we doing this?" ICU wait was immediately filled with my family and friends as we awaited the outcome.*

*Finally, after what seemed like days, Dr. Miller came in, found me and, at my request, told the whole waiting room (of friends) again--that Jim was in critical condition, he was able to clean him out as best as he could and his biggest fear was "the integrity of Jim's abdominal cavity" and the ability for it to "wake up." Essentially, Jim's intestinal cavity looked like a dead person's. A very somber, sad day. The next 48 hours would tell the story and Jim was again on a ventilator strapped to a zillion things in*

*ICU. Many were sure Jim would not make it as I looked around the room and I could see it in the faces of the medical team. I just kept the faith and kept wearing my cowboy boots, refusing to give up and remembering the angel that I firmly believe God sent.*

*At this point I quit writing so much in the journal (except for the medi- cal, clinical documentation) and started posting updates on my Facebook page because I have a lot of family who live in Texas and friends across the globe who follow me there. All I can say here is that I truly thought death was possible at this point. So did Dr. Miller who told me it was slim and critical and to be "prepared" for anything. That of course meant his death and funeral. I had refused to give up but the practical side of me knew I had to consider the possibility so I did organize a small group of close friends to help me should that become necessary. People were giving me hospice advice and cremation advice--very frightening to me. Thankfully, Jim kept fighting and so did I.*

*The next 6 days in ICU were just plain horrible. Jim was sedated, on the ventilator, losing weight and his medical team was worried about his nu- tritional status. Days blurred together and after so much trauma, I could only imagine the worst. Eventually they weaned him off the ventilator only to have to do a tracheostomy on him which would ensure oxygen flow without potential permanent damage to his vocal cords. He still could not breathe on his own and he couldn't communicate which was the most frustrating thing. He was too weak to write anything and could not even point to letters. The dilaudid drug was working on pain but doing strange things to Jim's mind. This was the worst period of darkness. We prayed, friends came and went and stayed close to me. My good friend from col- lege, JeanAnn Beckley came to town to be with me and I loved so much her uplifting visit. My sister was there whenever possible and my parents came and went. I lived mostly at the hospital. And I remember thinking how much I detest fluorescent lighting.*

*We were still in ICU on St. Patrick's day and I got some green and fun stuff for his room and gave all the RNs green stickers--anything normal was therapeutic for me. At this point Jim was having awful coughing spells and I had to suck crud out of his trach tube with a sucking thing they had hooked to his bed. We had now been in ICU--a second time--for 2 weeks and Jim was so very thin. He could not eat and had lost so much weight that he looked like a concentration camp survivor. That's the only thing I can tell you because it was true. His weight was down from his normal 190 to 142 lbs. I could see his bones and literally see him wasting away in the hospital bed.*

*Facebook continued to be my way of sharing and the whole world was praying for Jim. That must be why he was still here at this point.*

*March 18: Jim was moved to "step down" again on 3. He still could not eat, his abdominal cavity was still not "awake" and he desperately needed protein. I went back to sleeping in his room with him, and at 3:00 am we had to tie his hands to the bed as the was trying to pull out everything including his trach and oxygen. The sweet RN keeps calling him "Darlin" which we always said in Texas and I just love her for being so awesome. I am about at the end of my rope! Sweet RNs are good when you have had your limit, I promise! I got zero sleep and the next day friends came to take a day shift or two so that I could go home and shower.*

*Jim now had an NG tube (to pull bile out of his stomach) and could talk some but could not eat. The next few days were a nightmare and--as bad as Jim was--I asked Dr. Miller to see what he could do to order us back to 4-West. Finally we got back to room 423, happy to be where everyone knew us. Jim's chest x-ray looked better and Dr. Miller says he would remove the NG tube--a big deal for Jim. Jim remained highly agitated, hungry and thirsty and we could not leave him as he tried to climb out of his bed. Friends took a few nights of shifts as I had gone for 5-6 straight nights at the hospital at this point.*

*Life must go on and on Friday, March 20, Bryan toured the University of Memphis. Although he had been accepted at Mississippi State, he wanted to attend close to home given everything happening. So Bryan went on a tour of Memphis and loved it. Normally, where your kid goes to college is a big deal. I thought to myself, just get him in somewhere and we'll deal with it later if he wants to go elsewhere. When life and death knocks on your door, you do the best you can and I'm grateful for Bryan's intuition and family team efforts. Under normal circumstances, college visits and choices would be a big deal. Thankful for Bryan's wisdom and willingness to attend U of M.*

*I left the hospital to have lunch with Alys Drake and Bryan who met us there to tell us about his tour. I had only been gone from the hospital 30 minutes and I got a call from Jim's RN, Genetti, who told me Jim had ripped out his tracheostomy and oxygen and that respiratory and pulmonary had been paged to the room in case he could not breathe on his own. She tells me, "Stay put. We have this...I will call you right back." I ordered lunch but wanted to throw up but kept a good front for Bryan. In a few minutes Genetti called me to say Jim was breathing fine on his own and they don't need the tracheostomy anymore. Thank God for small steps and the great nurses at 4W.*

*We finished lunch and I took Bryan shopping for some desperately needed clothes and a pair of shoes. I got him two pair of khakis, a few shirts and some shoes. We then went back to the hospital where Bryan told Jim all about his day at U of M and his tour although Jim really wasn't fully comprehending.*

*March 21: Jim was being slowly weaned off pain meds and we were able to get him into a wheelchair with all of his machines on a pole that roll alongside. You need a course in "cord management" to help patients like Jim. I took him downstairs to the first floor so he could look out the window and see the Bradford Pear trees that were bloom-ing. He was weak and after only 5 minutes wanted to get back to his room. Hard to believe his stamina was reduced to a wheelchair ride for a few minutes. In the past 3 months, Jim has gone from a muscular, fit, strong man into a fragile, sick, skinny one but at least he's here. Baby steps and prayer.*

*March. 22: Bryan shot today in a Trap tournament and after that we all went to see Jim.*

*Days dragged by slowly...Jim was eating soft foods, practicing walking and having a tough time gaining any weight. March 26: Dr. Miller removed 2 drains and Jim had another CT scan which showed too much infection to leave the hospital. By this point, Jim had developed a bedsore, and although the RNs did a good job moving him often, it would be impossible not to develop one under Jim's circumstances. I bought a donut pillow for Jim to sit on as much as possible to relieve the bedsore pressure. Our friend Molly Polatty brought us a back pillow to use so Jim could sit up better in the bed...thankful for small blessings.*

*Days rolled by and we said goodbye to March and as April ushered in Spring, I told Jim that I could see light at the end of the tunnel. He said to keep telling him that.*

*April 1: As if we needed another complication, Dr. Miller reported that Jim has a "fistula"--hole in the small bowel which will keep him from eating. Dr. Miller was highly concerned with his nutritional status and says Jim was way behind. TPN and smoothies would continue but at this point, they would barely keep him going and the fistula must close and heal on its own. At this point, Jim cannot eat food until it does. It could take weeks. Jim's weight continues to decline along with his strength and stamina. His body is now "eating itself" and he is down to the low 140's.*

*Easter comes and goes and we spent it at the hospital as a family (and then we ate at the Sappenfields) grateful for Jim's life but weary of the fluorescent lights, pump beeps, cords and tubes. The next week passed without much progress but Jim was able to have smoothies which I got for him daily. He was getting thinner by the day and we just prayed hard that the fistula would close. I spent these days mostly at the hospital with my laptop and cell phone working when I needed to which was actually helpful.*

*I decided to host a "Healing Garden Party" in the Methodist prayer and healing garden for Jim, his medical team and our friends. Something positive to look forward to. We set the date for April 8th and the hospital and medical team approved it. It was fun and although Jim couldn't stay* long, we dressed him up and rolled him down to say hello to people he hadn't seen and show our gratitude for all of the support. I served wine, cheeses, fruits and water. It didn't last long but was uplifting to all and a way for me to thank many people. 4Memphis Magazine's Mark Ramirez came to take photos and we did a full page tribute to the Methodist team and friends in the magazine. If fact, that was helpful as many people still didn't know what had happened to Jim.

*April 10:* Dr. Miller thought that Jim could go home soon--even with everything going on but it meant a Herculean effort on my part. They did another CT to see if Jim was clear enough to leave and finally 4/13 we got released to head home. Home required daily TPN which was a 12-hour push of liquid nutrients through a PICC line he had which required me to administer every night. There was too much to go into but suffice it to say, I was going to have to be Jim's RN around the clock. The only good thing was that we were home.

So I shifted into high gear and did what I had to do: Flush PICC lines, empty ostomy bag, change dressings, charge the wound vac, administer TPN, put vitamins in the TPN bag with a syringe, monitor Jim's vitals, monitor Jim's nutritional intake, help him dress, empty urinals--you get the picture. I know there were days when I couldn't shower and often, I'd take a hot bath after I had Jim settled in bed, TPN going. With TPN, once it started (battery pump operated) he could not get out of bed for those 12 hours. Exhausted at this point would be an understatement! This was far worse than having a new baby or anything I have ever imagined.

This above routine lasted until I got a spontaneous (and much needed) break. I had committed to be a keynote speaker at the MO State Women's Bankers Association meeting and I went and took Mona Sappenfield with me. Jim's sister Julia and our kids took good care of Jim. I was only gone 2 days but it was a great break for me. Mona is a fun road trip companion, and I was speaking at a very upscale facility in the Lake of the Ozarks. We hit the spa as soon as we got there and managed to go back the second day following a keynote I gave to a crowded room of women bankers (Thank you to Trent Fleming for

*the kind recommendation). I spoke about "Women in High Gear" and
talked about the ultimate high gear test of having this current situation
happen. It was a therapeutic disruption and a great, legitimate reason
for me to go: I sold 250 books. I also met a woman (also a speaker) from
Texas named Honey Shelton who would prove to be a valuable business
contact for me in the future.*

*4/18: Bryan's Senior Prom: All the kids came over to our house for photos
and Jim helped Bryan get his tux on. It is hard to believe Bryan would
be graduating, and sad to me that we have had this trauma during what
would normally be happiest of times. The good news is that Jim is here
and that Bryan and Abby had stepped up and matured beyond what any
teen should have to. The kids looked so great in their formal duds and
we took photos of them and I think this was uplifting for us. Something
"normal."*

*4/28: Jim gained 2 more lbs and his weight was up to 150 lbs. He can
only walk using the walker and I have to carry everything. The fistula was
still draining (he had a drain and a bag which we measured daily) but it
seemed to be slowing. He still had to do the TPN daily which was probably the most confining and worst part of what I had to do--but critical
for Jim. The kids helped when they could, and were trained as backup in
case I couldn't get home in time or had an early meeting. I am working
and trying to take care of Jim. I don't see how single parents do it!*

*May 1: Deck days at the Howell's. I power sprayed and cleaned our deck
which took me two days but was great exercise and therapy. I loaded up my
bird feeders, bought some new cushions for our old chairs and an outdoor
rug from Pottery Barn that I found on sale. I was determined to make our
deck a happy one! We sat outside, watched gold finches, woodpeckers and
all kinds of birds from our deck. Jim still couldn't eat so we passed the days
doing what we have to, praying hard and were grateful for warm weather
and sunshine. Home care came twice per week, and worked with Jim to
empty his ostomy bag. While home care was there, I would often run to
Kroger or run to the drug store. It was like having a new baby--you can't
just leave. And we could not risk another fall.*

*May 12: Dr. Miller appointment concludes Jim's fistula was still there which was disappointing but at least Jim's weight was stable. You don't realize how enjoyable sharing a meal is until you cannot do it.*

*Things can change overnight. Woke up May 13 and Jim was not feeling well. He was coughing a lot and shivering with convulsions. I got him into a warm shower but that didn't help. I put him in bed with covers to see if he'd feel any better. The home health RN was scheduled for today and she arrived and Jim's fever was up a bit. Concerned, I sent Dr. Miller a text. We gave Jim Tylenol but at 5:30 PM on a gorgeous May afternoon, I texted Dr. Miller that Jim's fever has risen to 102.5. He texted me back "GET JIM TO THE ER STAT." He thought Jim's PICC line could possibly be infected.*

*Here we go again. I got him to the ER in my car (kids came with me) where more cultures were done and it's determined that Jim had an infected PICC line--a common thing apparently but dangerous in Jim's case. After several hours in ER, we finally got to 3 East at 12:30 AM. I got Jim settled and actually had to show the RNs there how to empty his ostomy bag as they weren't that familiar with it. I did it and headed home around 1:45 AM.*

*Again, I lined up school transportation for Abby (she wasn't happy but it was necessary) and of course Bryan drove himself. I cannot wait til Abby can drive herself.*

*5/14: Arrived at hospital and Jim was up talking to the RNs and I gave him a smoothie. He was on antibiotics and now out of danger from the PICC line--which would have been serious if not immediately addressed. They had IV antibiotics going and Dr. Miller said Jim was out of the danger zone again. I cannot believe how infection moves so quickly around the body.*

*Jim was doing better and in good hands on 4-West. I decided I would go downtown to my office, stay downtown a few nights and go to the Memphis in May BBQ festival where we had a team and I was entertaining clients.*

*It was a great break for me. Even Dr. Miller came down for some BBQ and I didn't realize how deprived I had been of some normal fun. With Jim back in the hospital, I didn't have to do the TPN, I was no longer tied to home and I could work some and sleep some. It was a glorious two days for me and a much needed break from the TPN. I hung out in out "Hog Wild" BBQ team booth with old friends and entertained some clients. Later our kids came down with friends and it was pure heaven for me to be surrounded by my kids and their friends.*

*May 18: CT scan showed fistula is GONE!!!! Jim could eat and eat he did! This meant no more damn TPN which was liberating for us all--mainly Jim but also for me. His first real food was hospital meatloaf and mashed potatoes which he said tasted great! I caught myself laughing as he previously had told dietary to quit bringing him "crap on trays." Amazing what you miss when you cannot have it--especially food. Dr. Miller is keeping Jim in the hospital to monitor his weight and also to get him ready for surgery #4--a skin graft to go over his open wound and get rid of the wound vac.*

*May 19: BRYAN HOWELL Graduation from Houston High School!! Jim could not attend but thanks to technology, he could watch from an app on the i-pad in the hospital. We all went and I am feeling physically so exhausted on top of this emotional moment of Bryan's life. I could not get home fast enough after graduation services...I needed a hot bath and a glass of red wine! Surgery was set for tomorrow and sleep came eventually but not the deep, restorative kind.*

*Wed. May 20: Alarm at 5:45 and time to go! Skin graft surgery day for Jim (surgery #4 in this ordeal) The graft would be put over his wound (no more wound vac) to help hold everything in until the FINAL major surgery (which we haven't had yet) to put Jim back together, reverse the ostomy and sew him up for the final time.*

*Our pastor, Will Jones, came in to pray with us (which he did often) and says "Lord, keep Jim in your hands during this Odyssey." I thought maybe "Dante's Inferno" would be more accurate so I read the book of Job in the Bible to try and make sense of it all. I remember a paper I wrote in a college religion class on the book of Job. Here we were living it in some ways! The only thing that helps me right now is to think of those who have also really suffered. I try and put my situation in better perspective when I think of those less fortunate. It's not what happens to you but how you handle what happens.*

*Surgery went well. Dr. Miller did the skin graft with help from his partner, Dr. McGee and the graft is like a band-aid to hold it all together. They took the skin from Jim's thigh like scraping a rectangle section of sod from a field. He has a big rectangular wound that will heal and be a big scar. That skin went over his wound like you would cut a piece of sod out and place it in the dirt. Jim will have to wear a custom made support around his abdomen that has a hole in it where the ostomy bag is. So shirtless, Jim's abdomen looks pretty awful I must say.*

*After another week or so in the hospital, Jim was finally released and home health is called back again to help him for the next 3 weeks. It is hard to believe May is gone!*

*June came and I took Abby and her friend Somer to the beach for 2 weeks (a trip I had pre-paid and could not get a refund for) while Jim stayed home with Bryan--recovering--with much help from home health and home PT. Bryan had a summer job anyway and he would be there at night with Jim. The vacation for me and Abby was pure heavenly bliss like you cannot imagine. At first I did feel very guilty leaving Jim, but got over that feeling once I passed from Mississippi to the Alabama state line. I felt my spirit lifting and I could almost smell the salt air! Before we got to the beach, we stopped in Mobile, AL to attend the wedding of Leslie Rouse. My Dad performed the ceremony and we spent fun times with the McFadden and Rouse families and saw old Mobile friends we love (Otts, Lutz, Adams, McFadden, Rowell, Wells, etc.). The wedding was in the church I grew up in where Dad was the senior pastor, Government Street Presbyterian Church. It was healing in high gear to be back in that church with my parents and our old friends. Abby and Somer loved attending the wedding and reception and I loved showing off my very tall and wonderful daughter. We said goodbye to my parents, checked out of the Battle House Hotel and loaded the car to head east towards our beach stay on 30-A.*

*We rode bikes, ate great food and I think I read 3--if not 4 books. Thanks to Facebook, an added bonus was spending my birthday with friends from Memphis (Patty and Tim) and my Chi O little sister Rhodes friend, Susan Stribling ("Strib") was there too and we saw each other twice! Loved that so much. My college friends, Strib and Jean Ann know me best and we have loved each other since 1982. Best friends are the best medicine.*

*It was a great break but honestly not nearly long enough! I could have stayed the whole summer. But, my business needed me, my family needed me and so soon we were back home resuming life.*

*Summer is flying by, and Jim is doing better, gaining weight, having in-home PT 3 x a week (that we are paying for) eating and learning how to be self sufficient again. Dr. Miller has cleared him to drive and re-sume "normal" (within confines) activities. The order of the day now is to continue to heal, get strong and rest up for the final surgery--12 months away--where Dr. Miller will reverse and correct it all--what should have been done right in the damn first place.*

*I am not writing much here in the journal but facebook has been great and has become my timeline for our lives. I have spent much time catching up on work and needing to re-tool my PR firm. I am also working non-stop it seems on getting Book #2 published. It's a bit of a challenge but will be so worth it. Last night I stayed up until 4 AM working because I just could not sleep.*

*Fall/Winter 2015: Jim has regular MD appointments to check the skin graft. We cannot plan anything until we know when the next big and final "put him back together surgery" will be. Our life seems to be on perma-hold and honestly, this is like adding insult to injury.*

*I am working as much as I can and have sold my office location to give us some cash flow and convenience. My office in my house will be better for us all as we face the final surgery which will again, require a lot of my time. I have never been so challenged in my life but I am getting through it and most of my clients have remained loyal. I have lost some business however, but that hasn't been all bad. I've had to slow down some and that has allowed me more rest, more focus on select clients and working more from home. The new book is also taking off and I am being asked to speak on it quite a bit. I need capacity to do that, and feel my life is shifting for the better! I pray for God to use me to help others and I am finalizing this next book, "Healing in High Gear." Writing is a coping mechanism and a way to capture what happened--if not for our children someday--but for others we can help.*

*I have to be honest and say that Jim's ostomy bag is a **big deal**. I don't know how people live with them and I have mad respect for people who do. Jim has had his now for 15 months and it prevents him (us) from many normal activities. He has to be home to empty it probably every 4-6 hours and we have had a few--not many--issues in public. I won't go into all the details here but it is honestly so limiting and Jim's abdominal cavity is still distorted and disfigured. We can't really travel, we can't get in the water (boat), we can't plan any vacations, we have to take supplies with us everywhere we go, etc. While we are very grateful Jim is alive, trauma that we have endured has certainly taken a toll. Our marriage has been truly tested--in about every way you can test it. When something this vulgar, traumatic and invasive happens to your spouse, it also happens to you. As a spouse, you share in the day to day living of the situation. I will say Jim handles it very well. I don't know if I would handle it as well as he has. Life is full of roses with sharp thorns. We are ready for our life back, more roses and less thorns.*

*May, 2016: The past 9 months have consisted of Jim healing, eating, exercising and getting strong enough for the next surgery which is now set for June 14, 2016 (Flag day--which I think is interesting given the current political landscape). Dr. Miller and Dr. Chandler (plastic surgeon) will go in, attach his colon, remove the "bag", pull his abdominal muscles back and sew him up. It will be MAJOR and recovery will last a few months. Dr. Miller expects that Jim to be in the hospital for 10 days and then home for about an eight week recovery.*

# CHAPTER 2

## Sepsis: The Masked Murderer

> "Sepsis is an insult to a surgeon"
> --ANONYMOUS

I had always heard of sepsis (and septic shock) but never in my wildest dreams would I believe I would come face to face with it multiple times. I call it the "masked murderer" because it is very hard to detect, moves very fast and can literally "mask"" itself as something else. Someone with sepsis may look like they have the flu at first. They may look like they are having a stroke or having respiratory problems. They may look like they have heart problems. You see, sepsis-caused by toxic leaking of waste into the body and blood stream-works mysteriously traveling around and shutting down systems and organs fast. The fatality rate is so high because most people either don't recognize it fast enough or waste valuable time treating something they "think" the symptoms reflect, but really aren't. Simply put, sepsis is the primary cause of death from infection. It is more common than heart attacks and claims as many lives as cancer (maybe more) yet many people still don't know much about it. Here are some statistics pulled from the Sepsis Alliance website www.sepsis.org

"In a study released in 2011, the Healthcare Cost and Utilization Project (H-CUP) identified 836,000 hospital discharges in 2009 where septicemia was a principal diagnosis, and 829,500 discharges where septicemia was a secondary diagnosis. The in-hospital mortality rates for each were 16.3% and 14.7%, respectively, totalling 258,204 deaths per year directly attributable to sepsis.

With more than 258,000 lives being lost per year, sepsis ranks as the third leading cause of death in the U.S. (after heart disease and cancer). Using data by the Centers for Disease Control and Prevention (CDC), sepsis would rank higher than chronic lower respiratory diseases, stroke, Alzheimer's disease, diabetes, and accidental deaths.

The same H-CUP report identified that there are more than 1.6 million cases of sepsis every year and survivors often face long-term effects post-sepsis, including amputations, anxiety, memory loss, chronic pain and fatigue, and more. Almost 60% of sepsis survivors experience worsened cognitive (mental) and/or physical function.

Many sepsis survivors also require rehospitalization. Over 62% of people who had a primary diagnosis of sepsis (the reason why they were hospitalized in the first place) who had to be readmitted to the hospital were rehospitalized within 30 days of first leaving the hospital. And among children, almost half who have had severe sepsis end up being hospitalized again. Sepsis is also the most expensive in-hospital condition in the U.S., costing more than $20 billion each year counting just acute care in-hospital costs."

In Jim's case the first surgeon, Dr. X, as well as the on-call doctor who released him missed it. The on-call team looked for heart issues while he was septic and we didn't know it. The only reason I was able to catch it and get him to the ER is due to my friend, a nurse anesthetist, Shannon. How I met Shannon is a funny story.

One day about four years ago now, I had to have a small cyst removed that required surgery and she was on the case. I was sitting in the waiting room before surgery when she popped her head out of the door to look at the cowboy boots I had on. I happened to be wearing my Texas boots that I had custom made with longhorns on them. Shannon literally opened the door, looked at my boots and then retreated back to the operating room (OR) area. A few seconds later, my surgeon popped her head out of the door to also look at my boots. I was thinking "what the heck is going on?" Later, as I rolled into surgery, Shannon introduced herself and told me she was a big OU fan (Oklahoma University) and that my boots were "terrible" as Texas is a big rival. The game was on and I was immediately loving the fun we were having. She said, "you know I'm the one that gets to put you under for this little operation so you'd better take those boots somewhere else." We laughed and soon the entire OR knew about my boots. When I came out of the surgery and was in recovery, my boots had been altered. The team had taped the OU logo over my longhorns as a joke. From that day on, Shannon and I became friends and soon, we were friends on Facebook. Working some in the medical field (I have PR clients who are physician groups) Shannon and I crossed paths some and we got to know one another outside of the OR. I believe God led me to her and somehow the cowboy boot thing must be a catalyst for finding good people. Anyway here is how Shannon played a key role in helping me save Jim (and in case you are wondering, the cyst they found was nothing but a small mass of nothing so no worries there).

Normally Shannon is in the OR during the day. However, that Monday-- when I tried to get Jim's Dr. (when he was septic) --I sent Shannon a text and told her Jim had fever. She called my phone immediately and said, "Amy, he could be septic. You have to get him to the ER now and tell them you think he's septic. Tell them to do an abdominal CT." After hearing those words, I did exactly that and she was exactly right. The abdominal CT showed that his colon was not attached and it was "raining sepsis" in his abdominal cavity. As previously stated, the ER doctor's words were "train wreck."

In Jim's case, the sepsis was a 10 on a scale of 1 to 10 (bad)--so much of it and it shut down his kidneys first. Kidneys shut down in order to protect other organs and they are usually the body's "first responders." Most people in Jim's condition would have died. The mortality rates for sepsis support this and we truly believe Jim is a "miracle man." Only God could have saved him and I think did, working His miracle through Dr. Miller.

Unfortunately there is not enough information available on sepsis that is shared often. You can find a lot of medical and clinical information online but as far as general awareness goes, we have a long road ahead. In my experiences with sepsis up close, I can tell you that the medical team--as good as they are-- missed it several times. If we don't make our first responders, ER teams and ICU teams more aware of sepsis, more people will continue to die. They die of sepsis but the ruled or claimed cause of death is often something else like heart failure, organ failure. The underlying "masked murderer" is sepsis or septic shock.

I will tell you another story--a recent one. A month ago, my Dad (approaching 80 years old) who is in relatively good health had a gallstone issue. He went to the hospital in pain and they sent him home to drink fluids but did not put him on any antibiotics. My Mom didn't call me when she took him in, and at the time, I thought it strange they released him and I questioned her about it and encouraged her to get an appointment with Dr. Miller, which she did.

For the next two days Mom took care of Dad at home while he threw up and continued to get worse. The next night at 11:30 p.m. my phone rang and it was Mom. She said, "I have called an ambulance for your Dad. I think he's having a heart attack or stroke." I hung up and literally flew over to their house in the pouring down rain to arrive to see the EMT's loading Dad into the ambulance. Mom told me they said it was stroke. Thinking about his gallstone issue my instincts kicked in, driven by my adrenaline high and I literally crawled up into the ambulance (while the EMTs were telling me to get out) to see and talk to Dad. I touched him and he was blazing hot. The EMTs said "we are taking him to St. Francis' stroke center." To that I said, "No. That is not going to work. You take him right now to his hospital, Methodist Germantown (also the closest) and treat him for sepsis. I don't think it's stroke, I think he's septic." The EMTs argued with me a bit more but I wasn't having it. I think Mom thought I was nuts but I told her if it was stroke, Methodist was just as good. I knew it wasn't a stroke. I knew deep down Dad was septic. I called Dr. Miller (God love that man) on his cell at midnight--which he answered--as Mom and I followed the ambulance to Methodist. Once Dad was in the ER, I asked the doctor there to start blood cultures for sepsis and made sure ER knew that Dr. Miller would be Dad's surgeon. I didn't want ER randomly assigning someone I didn't know. *Note: You never know when you will need surgery in an emergency situation so it is good to have one already selected in case you land in the ER. If you don't have one, they may assign one depending on circumstances. This experience has taught me that I wouldn't want "just any surgeon" operating on me for sure!* The ER doctor on call also thought Dad was having a stroke but we insisted they start looking for sepsis, especially given the gallstone issue. I just figured there was a connection.

Bingo. Dad's gallbladder was highly toxic and sure enough Dad was septic. Dad spent the rest of the night in ICU getting IV fluids and antibiotics. Dr. Miller arrived the next morning, and surgery was set to remove the gallbladder immediately. As it turned out, his gallbladder was gangrene. *It was confirmed that had Dad been treated for stroke, valuable time-which he didn't have-would have been wasted and the outcome would have been different.* Dad was in ICU and on a ventilator for a few days and finally as I write this has been released to go to rehab for a few weeks and ultimately home to expect a full recovery.

I believe God had His Hand in this. Had I not been through it all with Jim, I would have believed the EMTs (no blame to them at all--they were doing their jobs) and would have never questioned what would have turned out to be the entirely wrong diagnosis. Sepsis is the dark, masked murderer. Two things helped me know it was not stroke:

- God would never take my Dad by stroke: I kept praying while I was standing in the rain arguing with the EMTs. I said "Please Dear God, tell me what to do, I know you would never take my Dad this way..." Dad is a retired Presbyterian Minister who has been a faithful servant of Christ and I just knew this was not the end.
- Dad had fever. As I crawled up into the ambulance to touch him and when I felt his forehead, I knew. He was blazing hot. Fever is a sign of infection and sepsis--this was my sign.

I know that God is faithful and I know that my Dad will pass someday (but not soon) but I knew it wasn't going to be in a thunderstorm in the back of an ambulance in a hospital we don't know. We don't know God's plan but I would guess my Dad will pass peacefully, when it's time and when my Mom is tired of him--ok, not really. My Dad is a big practical joker and he loves humor. He always tells Mom, me and my two sisters to just "bury me under the driveway so you all can just keep on running over me." Keeping a sense of humor-even in the darkness-is key.

## Signs of Sepsis

Slurred speech
Extreme shivering and muscle pain
Passing no urine in a day
I feel like I might die
Skin issues (discolored, rash)

Other signs of sepsis we noticed in our cases mimic the flu: fever, extremely low blood pressure and pain.

## What to do if you suspect sepsis & about sepsis

- Immediately get to the ER and tell them you think it could be sepsis (tell medical team to start blood cultures, give IV fluids and antibiotics and be adamant)
- Call the best surgeon you can--sepsis usually requires immediate surgery
- Prepare for the worst: kidney failure, ICU, and multiple complications
- Call other specialists you know and ask them to review medical case
- Don't be afraid to ask questions about updates on vital signs
- Don't leave your patient alone--even in the hospital
- Monitor closely blood pressure, heart rate, blood tests
- Know that sepsis can move around and is difficult to treat sometimes
- Prepare for a long recovery and possible complications/other issues
- Sepsis is painful and weakens patients drastically and quickly
- Sepsis triggers something in the brain that causes confusion and memory function--impacts cognitive function

Anyone who knows me knows how much I love Twitter. It's a fantastic tool for sharing information and doing research. I have found a few great resources: The Sepsis Alliance at www.sepsis.org in North America and Dr. Ron Daniels--founder and CEO of UK Sepsis Trust (a charity based in the UK). Dr. Daniels is known as the "sepsis six guy" and travels the world raising funds and awareness of sepsis. If you want more information, look at www.

sepsistrust.org and you will find great information there. *The sepsis six are his guidelines for the six immediate things the medical team must do when a patient is septic: Give oxygen, take blood cultures (and cultures take time to grow), give IV antibiotics, start IV fluid resuscitation, check lactate, monitor urine output.*

Sepsis is something that I believe deserves much more attention in the media and across the board in general. And just as a point of information, the month of September is "Sepsis Awareness month" and the color is any shade of orange. I think hospitals should light up their facilities in orange during the month of September and implement an awareness campaign to educate the general public on the danger of sepsis.

Obviously EMT's and first responders need more training. I hope this book will help shed light on the killer called sepsis. Further, we must do more to ensure successful surgical outcomes that don't include patients getting septic.

# CHAPTER 3

## When Tragedy Strikes: Shifting into High Gear Action

> "Visions without actions are hallucinations"
> --Dr. Michael Kami

don't do well in the "pause" mode. Maybe it's because I believe you must always be moving forward in your life, learning, growing, seeking. This is not to say being still to listen and absorb is not important. What I'm talking about is not becoming paralyzed or "frozen" when something bad happens. I think it is human nature to want to go bury your head in the sand, but that is just delaying the inevitable and creating even more problems. One of the reasons for writing this book is because I want to share my story with other spouses and family members and encourage and inspire them into the right action and "high gear thinking."

What is "high gear?" High gear is a state of mind that when reached, can drive you into positive action and achievable results. I have written several books (noted in the back of this one) about high gear and being "in high gear." High gear is not the same for everyone, but you can find yours by deliberately choosing to stand up to challenges, evaluate a situation at face value and act on it to produce necessary outcomes. You have choices! Even in the darkest hours, you have choices. Doing nothing or becoming paralyzed and unable to act is, in itself, a choice. And you must not take what the medical team says as always accurate. While they are usually correct-and trained to be-you must question a diagnosis and request conclusive tests that prove accuracy.

Never in a million (ok, zillion) years would I have allowed that first surgeon to do Jim's surgery back in Jan. of 2015 had I known what would follow. That's why the old saying goes that hindsight is 20/20. You cannot turn back time nor can you wish for a different outcome. Looking back too long is wasted time and energy. And time is a non-renewable resource you cannot get more of so don't waste it! You must deal with the cards on the table--the situation you are in now, and figure out the best strategy to improve your situation. You must look at facts only and try to suppress emotions--difficult as that may be.

When we raced Jim to the ER for that first time when he was full of sepsis, we all thought he would die. I could see it in the faces of the entire ER team and thankfully, their honesty prepared me for the worst. It helps that I do crisis communications and PR and maybe my training and experience helped me view my situation as I would from the outside. High gear for me meant I had to remove my emotional state from the current situation and think about how to help Jim. I told myself it would be like trying to save a client from a bad story in the press. It helped me focus on what to do. ACTION was needed. Here was Jim laying in the ER and later ICU literally on his deathbed. After thinking about it, I knew quickly how to help him.

Now this all happened so fast that looking back, I realized I was completely alone in that ER and ICU. I was so focused on Jim that I hadn't had time to tell anyone we were in the hospital nor how bad it was. Upon reflection, I believe this was a gift. Being alone allowed me to think and develop a strategy and action plan. It also allowed me to focus on what the medical team was telling me minute by minute--none of which was good.

I powered up my laptop and crafted an email to the CEO of the hospital we were in, Mr. William Kenley, CEO of Methodist Le Bonheur Germantown Hospital. I did not know him but my plan was to get to know him. My email summarized what had happened to Jim, the status of his critical condition, and my total lack of confidence in the first surgeon, Dr. X. Further, I told him that I wanted him removed from Jim's case, and a new surgeon brought on. Not only had I lost confidence in his surgical skills but I knew he was not responsive and had no "sense of urgency" on Jim's case. I suspected Jim might need additional surgery (4 more as it turned out) and I knew we had to change horses fast if we were in for the long ride. I ended the email by saying if we didn't do this, I was sure Jim would die and that I would be waiting in ICU to get this process rolling.

Mr. Kenley answered me the next day (my email was after midnight) early and Dr. Paul Douthitt, Chief Medical Director, came down to meet me with the appropriate paperwork for the requested changes. I have already told you what happened in chapter 1 so I will not repeat it.

The point is--while it is rare to have a surgeon removed from an active case--it was necessary. Convincing the hospital to review it fast and securing their support to do so was essential. The other thing I did that helped was call all the fine doctors I knew and Jim's other doctors to help me figure it out. After a new surgeon took Jim's case (Dr. Mark Miller), it became a team effort to save Jim with Miller leading the charge--in his **cowboy boots**, I might add. Dr. Miller is the type of surgeon and person who is confident but not to the point of being so arrogant that other opinions don't matter. His "team" approach involving other specialists allowed for the best results for Jim. Dr. Miller also listens to the nurses who--in my opinion and experience--often know as much (or more) about the status of the patients than the doctors do. And they spend the most time with the patients so **the best doctors will listen to the nurses.**

When you are in a crisis--medical or otherwise--you must review facts and you must get the best help you can using the resources you have. I did not know Mr. Kenley but I did know others in the administration who knew him. What I was counting on was doctors and friends in my network to have my back and vouch that I was not some crazy person upset about something trivial that happened in a surgery. There are a lot of crazies out there and it helps if you aren't one of them. *Stay calm and wear cowboy boots!*

High gear also means communicating to your network when you need something. You can't think of everything so it helps to surround yourself with smart friends and people who can think of things you may forget. A lot of the doctors who are our friends asked questions that helped me ask questions. If you don't know how to advocate or think in high gear, you can get someone who can and does.

## Before Any Surgery

Before any surgery, get your ducks in a row. Know where legal papers are, get the proper documents in place (living will, etc) and ask yourself this question: what if the patient goes into distress, a coma, or has to be sedated for an extended period of time? Are you ready to advocate? Do you know what the patient's wishes are? Could you make the tough decisions if your patient could not talk or communicate?

The state of TN is currently undergoing an awareness campaign that stresses the importance of "end of life" discussions and making wishes known. The clinical term is "advanced care directives" and you will hear about this more if you are in the hospital for an extended stay.

While nobody wants to have this "talk," it is important that we all do. We are all headed to the ultimate final destination so why not plan for that! I am working now with "Healthy Shelby" on a statewide private/public effort to promote awareness of families talking about end of life wishes. There is a lot about this at this website and www.theconversationproject.org.

Here in Memphis and across the state of TN, we are working collaboratively with partners, hospitals, insurance providers, etc. to help promote the importance of talking about wishes. Physicians are now being reimbursed for talking to their patients about end of life care (advanced care directives) as they are usually in the best position to have the conversation. We (Memphis, Nashville, Chattanooga and Knoxville hospitals and providers) are launching a statewide, public awareness campaign this year and our website will be live by the time this book is out. Shout out to Donna Abney, Patti Smith and Nancy Averwater for getting me involved in this important campaign. And I love meeting all the passionate, committed people across the state working on this important educational and awareness campaign.

*Talking is very important when a loved one is facing any type of invasive surgery.* Most people think "the talk" is for when you get old. Let me be your example of how important it is to know what your loved ones would want and to get it in writing--at any age! Accidents happen, bad surgery outcomes happen...don't wait! Talk now! Then act.

When Jim went in for the first surgery, we never expected the outcome we got. Thankfully, I knew (because we had talked about it) that Jim would never want to live if he could not be restored fully to his normal health. He told me he never wanted to be on long term dialysis or a ventilator (which he was but only temporarily). While I was certainly not "ready" to make medical decisions for him (like changing surgeons, etc) here we were and I was having to think and act for him. So, before any surgery do these things:

NUMBER 1 and most important: **Make darn sure you know your surgeon and their track record, reputation, and ability.** If you want to know about a surgeon, just ask the nurses. They know. Do not ever let a surgeon you do not know operate on you if at all possible. Do not sign your authorization for surgery without knowing what you are signing and who the surgeon will be.

- Get financials in order and let your spouse or family member know where things are and what passwords are if you pay bills online
- KNOW THE PATIENT'S SOCIAL SECURITY NUMBER! Good grief, you have to write it on just about every form there is!
- Pre-pay any household bills if you can for a month which gives you peace of mind if something goes wrong (and keep in mind you have to take care of someone following a surgery so there is not much time for other duties)

- Tell other medical specialists about the surgery and have them "clear" the patient (you would think that would be protocol but it's not. Dr. X didn't see any need for Jim to consult with primary care, cardiology, etc--I should have known this was not right but I had no idea at the time, and I trusted-wrongly-the surgeon)
- Have a "back up" surgeon: who would you want if you had to change surgeons? It's rare for a surgeon to be removed from an active case. In our case, it was life or death.
- Make a list of all medicines and prescriptions the patient takes and make about 100 copies of the list to keep with you
- Make sure all insurance premiums have been paid prior to surgery (our premiums are now on auto draft so we don't miss any and are not late)
- Make sure your spouse or advocate has access (legally) to bank accounts
- Have the conversation about "what if" and talk about worst case outcomes because you never know and they do happen; if you have an advanced care directive plan or living will, anything documented supporting your wishes, have it with you and give it to your family
- If you have a large estate or complex financial situation, seek legal counsel before surgery
- Let your banker, financial advisor and lawyer know about the surgery and ask them for recommendations if needed (transfer cash, etc). In our case, Jim was sedated for so long that I had to pay a large tax bill and turned to my advisors to help me get that done
- Talk about financials and loss of income--in our case Jim was unable to work for an extensive amount of time. That adds extra pressure and stress to any family.
- Make a list of what you would need if your patient landed in a long term hospital or recovery situation (who pays bills, who cuts grass, what are the household issues, child care issues, how would you function if your patient couldn't do anything for you or your household for months?)
- Get a lot of rest before surgery. I wish we had thought about taking a good, long vacation somewhere warm and sunny prior to Jim's surgery--at least I would have been rested and tan facing the hell we faced!

Nobody signs up to be in a hospital for 90+ days. When and if you ever do have to stay, you need to be ready for a lot of stressful days. I don't know how I did it looking back, but as John Wayne said, "Courage is being scared to death but saddling up anyway." You don't have a choice so you do what you have to do.

## High Gear Tips for extensive hospital stays

--You must ask questions and get people with you to ask them
--Think for yourself and trust your gut
--Move fast: be decisive when time is running out
--Call friends who have been through something and get input/advice
--Listen carefully to the medical team members and write down what they say
--Be the squeaky wheel if something is wrong
--Document while in the hospital and keep a daily journal --put in as many details possible
--Understand that doctors are human and make mistakes; watch your patient closely
--Ask for help when you need it
--Surround yourself with support but limit visitors for patient
--If you don't have any support (friends or family) ask the hospital chaplain to find someone
--read scripture and daily devotionals and ask God for strength

And the best doctors will let you "vent" and I remember one night I was standing outside in my driveway when Dr. Steve Threlkeld (same class with me undergrad at Rhodes College) called me when Jim was in ICU and not ok. The medical team had missed a round of antibiotics and I was not happy. When Dr. Threlkeld called me (and I call him Steve), I think I pretty much gave him a piece of my mind and guess what? He took it like the gentleman he is, reassured me, stayed on the phone with me and made me feel better. I said "OK, Steve, I'm not talking to you as a doctor, I'm talking to you as a classmate and friend and I'm pissed." He was awesome. He and his brother took amazing care of Jim and I cannot be more grateful. My point is that sometimes honesty and tough conversations happen. Anger and frustration are a normal part (and healthy) of what we went through. I think I was able to use that anger productively to get my points across and stand my ground to help Jim. The best physicians will listen to you vent and help you through it.

If you are in a hospital with a loved one or in a similar situation, what can you add to this list? Write it down in the margins of this book and refer to it. What example of high gear are you seeing in some of the medical staff? Your spouse?

I can tell you that Jim Howell is in high gear. There is nobody tougher who can beat sepsis multiple times. His high gear fight is what got him through it. And knowing he was literally fighting for his life is what got me and our family through it.

# CHAPTER 4

## Stress on the Caregivers: Support systems, Friends and Coping Tools

> "I just don't have time for the nervous
> breakdown I deserve…"
>
> --SOMETHING TO TALK ABOUT (ONE OF MY FAVORITE MOVIES)

At first, when Jim was so critical--to be honest--I didn't want to see anyone except our children. Understandably, Jim was strapped to machines and at death's door and what goes through your mind at the time is almost beyond imagination. What I kept thinking was this, "just a week ago Jim was healthy and working out." Things can change at the slice of a surgical instrument. So there I was, alone in ICU with my husband unable to communicate. Scary moments you should not have to face alone.

Thanks to texting and social media sites such as Facebook, it didn't take long for word to get out that Jim was in ICU and in trouble. People came in herds and I was so grateful to see smiling faces even in the midst of devastating circumstances. Friends brought food up to the ICU waiting area which felt like my home away from home. Days passed and friends stayed by me and our family, praying hard, buying gift cards for our kids (I wasn't home to cook), bringing gift baskets and flowers, taking me out to eat or to get away from the hospital for a spell, etc.

My sisters were there by my side and one even came from South Carolina to stay with me at the hospital. My college best bud, Jean Ann Beckley, flew from Charleston to come stay a few days and just "be" with me. My Memphis friends were steadfast, visiting almost daily to cheer me up. Our ministers from our church came often, praying for us and leaving notes if Jim was out for dialysis or tests.

Never underestimate the support of friends, family and churches. I think Jim was on every prayer list across the city if not country. People who don't even know us were praying for us when they heard Jim's story. People who follow me on Twitter and Facebook were sending me messages of hope and healing.

Many people use "Caringbridge" to post updates on critical loved ones. I decided not to because I already had 'built my tribe' on Facebook--friends across the globe and extended family in Alabama, South Carolina and Texas. At first, I was hesitant about posting, but as time went on, Jim became more critical and I decided it was the best way to get information out. My phone was blowing up and I couldn't answer every text. I wanted a strategy for updating so I decided that a daily "Jim Howell update" would be how I would do it. So much changed with Jim that it was up, down, up, down. One update would capture a 24-hour progress report. And my close friends were by my side, often texting others to let them know Jim's status. Soon it seemed everyone knew to check Facebook and that was key for me.

I cannot tell you the comfort I got from reading all of the Facebook comments after a status report. I realize some people don't want to comment because they don't want to be notified of all the updates, but let me tell you I read each comment over and over, and it helped me. I could feel the love through Facebook friends and that lifted me. Posting was easier than talking on the phone (I was exhausted--physically, mentally, emotionally) and people could pray for specific things about Jim. I would post "pray for his kidneys to work," and people would pray for that. Later I would post "pray for his fistula to close," and people prayed for that. People became so interested in Jim that I had friends tell me, "I never go on Facebook but now I am daily to check your page." If I missed a post or waited too long to post, I would start getting texts from people asking "how is Jim?" So Facebook is a great tool to use in high gear healing for me. I know it's not for everyone, but it worked and became an extended support system for our family.

The other thing that happens is when someone like Jim has so many issues, there was something every minute that I had to attend to. The medical team was like a revolving door taking care of Jim's many issues. Due to his critical and often extreme condition, he didn't have just one doctor. He had an army of them--each specialist looking at something different. As an advocate, my focus had to be on what the team was saying, tests, dialysis, medications, wound care, etc. I needed to be the quarterback communicating with the team. I did not have time (or energy) to talk to other people and my focus was completely on Jim.

When something happens, the spotlight is on the patient--as it should be. However, there needs to be more focus on the emotional, physical, mental and financial wellness of the caregivers out there. As a caregiver, I can tell you that it is one of the most challenging and difficult things--for many reasons--that you can ever do. And guess what? You never know when this role is forced on you. It's not something you choose. Now I would not be being honest with you if I said "everything is fine and high gear means you just suck it up and move." There are times when I was certainly not in high gear. I am writing this to tell you that as one who is normally strong and in forward gear, there were days I was not and I still have those days. That is normal y'all. What happens when you find yourself in the caregiver role is that you basically lose yourself for the sake of taking care of others. In my case, it meant taking care of Jim, my kids, my business, my employees (who actually helped take care of me too) and how in the world do you do it? It's like putting everything into the blender and pressing start. You just do it. You do it because you don't have another choice. Instead, I helped myself by thinking about people in worse situations. I seriously thought a lot about the Holocaust and concentration camps, torture, ISIS and mass shootings, and being in prison. That helped my perspective--thinking about people who suffered far more.

Here are some of the things I did to cope and I hope you find these help-ful. They are not manufactured, they are really things I did--some of which I haven't told anyone about.

**Diet**: at first, I could not eat. Later, I made up for it and tried to eat good foods that gave me nourishment and strength. I will never forget Leslie & Peter Schutt bringing me fresh and incredible home grown spinach. I tried to eat a steak now and then and took my vitamins. Believe it or not, after all those days in the hospital, I never once caught a cold or got the flu. (Note: You can find Peter Schutt's spinach at his new midtown store, The Curb).

**Rest**: I believe it has taken me **one full year** to catch up on lost sleep but I took long naps often when I could even when I knew I should be working. I remember thinking "Ok Amy, you can't work if you're dead." Rest when you can and often. I think I'm still catching up!

**Wine, Dine & Friends:** I drank wine (good wine--never bad wine) with dinners with my girlfriends often. When you are so stressed, upset and bound to the hospital all day and night, going out to dinner was something I looked forward to. Thank you to my friends who brought me wine (and yes, we snuck it into the hospital waiting area sometimes, especially on weekends) and helped me through it. I remember one night me and Alys Drake went to Erling Jensen's to eat and sweet Erling wouldn't let us pay for our dinner. I remember going to Mona Sappenfield's house because she lives so close to Methodist and I could get a break without going all the way home! She would sit me down and serve me wine and something good to eat.

One night--after dinner with friends I got home to find a wild, stray cat cornered by our great german shepherd, Grace (her full name is Amazing Grace given to her by her breeder). The cat--wrongly--had selected our yard to trespass in, and in light speed, Grace saw me pull into the driveway and pro-ceeded to grab the cat with her powerful jaw, snap the cat's neck, killing it on impact (the cat felt nothing) and--though sorry for the loss of any animal--this did not really bother me. Grace proceeded to drop the dead cat at my feet with her tail high as if to say, "look Mom, I got it!" For some reason this seemed crazy and comical to me in the moment. If I had not been at dinner with friends and happy, I might have seriously had a meltdown. We put the dead, wild cat in a bag and in the trash. The next day at the hospital when the kids were leaving, my dad shouted, "be sure to put all dead cats in the trash."--again, humor. When a human life hangs in the balance, it certainly puts things into perspective. Humor is important too.

**Writing**: I wrote in my computer diary every single day, and I also worked on book number two (***Students in High Gear*** now on Amazon) which was like a light at the end of the tunnel for me. Poor Anne Gallaher had to endure a co-author who was--justifiably--not herself! Thank you Anne for your kindness and patience as we finished the book! The wait was worth it, and I am so proud of our accomplishment and ever grateful for your friendship.

**Screaming and crying**: One night Bryan came to get me out of the driveway where I had gone to let a few screams out after I just couldn't hold them in after getting a call from one of the doctors. My sweet children took good care of their Mom I'm telling you. Bryan put his arm around me and led me back into the house. I did feel better but the neighbors did call the police who searched our neighborhood for a few hours. I didn't care. I cried some too but mostly prayed hard.

**Counseling**: In addition to talking to ministers and visiting chaplains, I did seek professional counseling. It helped some, but mostly validated that I was normal. My counselor told me I should be treated for "PTSD" for what I had seen and been through. The main thing she did was confirm that I was on a good track and had solid coping mechanisms and a good support system.

**Antidepressants**: I recommend them. I was on them for hot flashes a few years ago and got back on them for this stretch of life. I think my family is the main beneficiary of them but they help a lot and I don't feel guilty or ashamed of telling you this. I'm not superwoman although I do have a cape!

**Focus forward:** I got tired of hearing these words: "Baby steps." It's true. Move forward but take small steps and don't put too much pressure on yourself! Plan things to look forward to even if it's a simple dinner with a friend. The simple things are the best anyway.

**Know you will never be the same again:** Just like having a baby changes everything, being a caregiver in a stressful situation (especially if it is your spouse) will permanently change you, hopefully for the better, but expect a few rough patches along the road. Everything will look different through your new lens of whatever trauma you have experienced. For me, now trivial things, silly things, material things really don't matter and I have found I have no patience for them. Keep in mind this will also test and alter your friendships, and can impact key relationships in your life. Real friendships will endure everything you go through. Friendships based on less will become so. Know that this is normal and be at peace with it. I am blessed with good friends and a new perspective.

It isn't easy being a caregiver and everyone is so focused on the patient. Even today, as we are well into year two of this ongoing medical nightmare for Jim, everyone asks me "How's Jim?" Of course they do! That is normal. Caregivers need to be asked how they are as well, and caregivers have to take care of themselves. They have to rest, eat, sleep, get a massage, get exercise, etc. to carry on. It requires great physical strength to be a caregiver. It also takes emotional and mental stamina--especially if it is your spouse. Some days you are just so worn out and often to the point of not being able to sleep.

The good news for me is that Jim realizes what I have had to do and we talk about it often. I appreciate the fact that he appreciates everything I did and am doing. I can see how a marriage would not survive something like what we have survived. It is hard enough to be married in ideal situations. Often, when a crisis like this occurs, you have added stresses in physical, financial, medical and emotional areas. I can say it really depends on how you handle it and the faith that you must lean on daily. I will admit it and tell you honestly that our marriage has been tested in every single way: physically (sexually), emotionally, mentally and financially. High gear means working through it and not giving up on each other. High gear also means seeing the light at the end of the very dark tunnel and knowing it's not a train. Our marriage is shifting to a new phase--one based on gratitude, strength and faith.

If you are a caregiver and a breadwinner for your family like I have been, you must also resist the temptation to resent your position and further resent other people going about their happy, normal lives. At times--when we were in the middle of the storm--some friends would take trips to luxurious places and I would think "wow, I'll never get to do that." You simply cannot allow yourself to get so inwardly focused that you become bitter or envious. Jealousy is the worst sin. It will destroy relationships, families and anything that it can. Don't be that person. Yes, you deserve a luxurious trip too. But remember this: nobody can relate to what you have been through unless they have and most have not--thankfully. When you are a caregiver, I think it is helpful to talk to those who actually have been in those same shoes. Fortunately, none of my friends (except for one) have really had something like what happened to Jim in their own lives. Yes, people die but let me tell you something: in some cases, death can be easier. I didn't say better, I said easier.

Don't blame people for seeming "clueless" and "oblivious" to what you are experiencing. They simply don't have the depth of experience that gives them any true, relatable perspective. Instead, focus your mind, thoughts, prayers and energy on forward progress, restorative and positive healing. Focus on a mindful willingness to overcome and be positive. Seek friends that are positive. I sometimes like to "think myself into a winning situation" and I find it works. I literally visualize myself being happy and positive and sharing that with those who feel the same.

Further, trauma like what we experienced will--after some time--alter your friendships and perspective. I want to use this experience to help others and be there for my real friends as a friend should be. Looking back, I have asked myself questions challenging the real meaning of friendship. It has become very clear to me what is really important in a friendship, and the main thing I take from all of what happened is to BE a friend to others in the way I would want my friends to be to me.

You also must forgive your friends for what they don't know, and you have to forgive yourself for letting go. This has been a very personal journey--one that I hope will be used to hasten in only the best of friends with the best of intentions.

I do have one friend (you know who you are) who has been through "it" including surgeries like Jim's. This friend is a hero and has been a great inspiration to me and we are praying for her daily.

A few other things I did to cope in the midst of the really bad times:

--used my "alone" status to focus on renewed priorities in my life and work
--prayed often leaning on God to be in charge
--watched uplifting movies (I still refuse to watch sad dramas) to escape
--took long walks--often around the hospital and in my neighborhood
--got a few facials at Mona Sappenfield's incredible spa
--cooked a few times for my teens and their awesome friends (kids cheer me up)
--put a fire in my fireplace any night I was home
--worked on writing and client projects--a great diversion and made me feel productive
--fed the birds in my backyard and enjoyed their beauty

If you have never had to be a caregiver, count your blessings. And I have huge respect for those who choose a profession in caregiving. While each situation is different and each patient has different circumstances and needs, the chore itself is similar. I think I should print some bumper stickers that say "Hug a Caregiver" and put them at every hospital and nursing home in America! If you have never been one, hopefully you won't have to be, but there is a good chance you will. I hope these tips help you.

# How to help caregivers

--pray for them and with them
--listen to them--let them talk it out
--don't try and give them advice or tell them about your experience unless you have had theirs'
--don't take it personally if they lash out or are not themselves
--bring food (gift cards are better--often times food gets thrown out) but don't just show up
--start a fund or donate to them--a lot of things are not covered by insurance
--help advocate for them if you see they cannot

--help them with information or contacts that could help

--sit with them at the hospital but make sure that's what they want: ask

--don't be offended if they tell you "it's not a good time"

--relieve them at the hospital so they can get a break

--help with family needs (drive carpool, feed dogs, etc)

--send them notes of encouragement and scripture

--feed their medical team

--don't make it all about YOU--It's about them right now

--say things like "I don't know how you do it" or "you are a warrior" or "you are inspiring"

I remember one day I got home to find a note in my mail with a card from Patti Clauss that just said "You ROCK" signed, "I love you." —very helpful and comforting.

Can you add to this list? What would you want from a support group if you were caring for someone?

# CHAPTER 5

## Financial Matters

> "We make a living by what we get...but
> we make a life by what we give."
> --WINSTON CHURCHILL

When a tragedy of this scale happens to a family--and a chief earner can no longer work--high gear shifting into financial strategy is necessary. In our case, Jim was in the process of interviewing for a new job, being offered a job, and was doing consulting work. Post surgery, Jim obviously could not accept that job much less work for months on end. This--is in and of itself--a hardship. As I write this we are making some decisions with respect to savings and our retirement that we were hoping to delay. We have sold some assets and are trying hard to balance our family financial needs. I must say, I am proud of what we have been able to do and how we've done it.

Initially, a medical fund was established at first by friends and family and we were able to raise funds from generous friends and family for some immediate needs (Huge thank you to those who donated--we love you all). When something happens like what happened to us, a family needs cash. Insurance only pays so much and medical bills are mind-blowing. There are also "out of network" costs such as physical therapy and other services you may need that come out of your pocket. In our case, we had home health but insurance only covered so much. If you need additional help at home with a patient, you must private pay for that.

Additionally, as Jim is the accountant in the family, he was paying bills so one of my immediate challenges was to find out where everything was (on his computer) and pay bills. One tip for everyone: **Before any surgery of any kind, make sure your spouse or family member knows where financial information is and passwords to your computer.** We do a lot online and I had trouble finally getting all of our passwords for different accounts. So much of the initial illness had Jim under sedation and communicating with him was often impossible.

In most cases, the hospital will work with you to negotiate financial issues and navigate through bills. It is also important to cross reference your EOB's (explanation of benefits) with medical records. Insurance companies and hospitals make errors and it is important to review them often and document information. You may be paying for something you do not owe.

The hospital can also advocate for you with insurance companies and thankfully, the Methodist team did just that. At one point the insurance company had rejected a "wound vac" which Jim had to have so the hospital team had to convince them he really needed it.

Although there have been many advances in clinical care, our national healthcare system has a long way to go. Hopefully we will have higher gear leadership that will focus on prevention, education and access. In a day where we have the most technology and information possible, we should have the best access to care.

# High gear tips for dealing with the financial side of illness

--Get some help if you can (financial planner, accountant, banker, lawyer)
--Make a list of immediate bills owed, where funds are, get your arms around current status
--Don't panic--easier said than done but true
--Notify anyone you owe of your medical status and ask for an extension in writing

--Do accept donations graciously from a medical fund and get family to start and promote it;
Everyone wants to bring you food and that's what we do in the south, but if everyone would spend that $30 it takes to deliver a meal and start a fund, that's truly helpful. We had a friend call and say "how much is an RN for a week, I want to pay for that." Great way to help a family.

--Meet with your banker! My banker is a good friend, Dana Burkett, and she helped me navigate accounts and transfer funds when needed. Your banker can help you pay bills help you solve problems and think through immediate financial issues

--Go on a budget and immediately look for expenses to cut from family budget

--Pray hard and try to stay positive that things will work out even if it means a change in your financial status

--Understand that something like this is "life changing" and that you and your family may never be in the same position you were before; This is where financial planning is important

--Make you teenagers work: In our case, Bryan had a job and still does which helps offset some of his expenses; As I write this now, Abby has turned 16 and also has a job. When tragedy strikes, the high gear family gets everyone pulling in the same direction

Finally, nobody ever expects something to happen to them like what happened to Jim. Thankfully, Jim and I had been very conservative and had tried to save and pay off debt over the past decade before this happened. I give a lot of credit to my banker Dana who helped us do some planning to position us for better retirement goals. We had no idea how much we'd need it at the time we executed the plan. The fact that we were not "leveraged" when this happened is why we have not lost everything we have. At a minimum, this will be a two to three year "crisis" when it is all said and done, and you have to be financially ready for something when and if it comes. We hope to recover fully but from a financial standpoint, we may never. Time will tell.

I would recommend to anyone reading this that you try and get out of any debt if you can, be very conservative and save as much as you can--if you can.

Our lives have been turned upside down and while it is not fair that this happened, it did happen. Nobody deserves what we are going through but sitting back and complaining does no good. Instead, we embrace our new status of "poorer but alive." I never really, fully appreciated the "Give us this day our daily bread" until now. It really is true. There is no promise of tomorrow and we all must live with our realities of today. We have made family decisions to adjust and have altered some things to weather this unimaginable storm.

# CHAPTER 6

## Dealing with Hospitals, Medical Teams, Surgeons

> "Maybe one day when I hear 'breakfast in
> bed' I won't think of a hospital room."
> --ME

There is no "how to" playbook to use when it comes to dealing with complex, devastating medical illnesses and everyone you must communicate with. That is why I am writing this from personal experience in hopes that it can help others who find themselves in a similar situation. When it comes to navigating the web of a hospital system, you must think in high gear and arm yourself with facts and information. I have already described the situation we encountered during the first trip to ICU. What I haven't described is the approach I took and why I knew it could work.

During a crisis, you must keep calm. Your tone and attitude from the beginning can set the pace and agenda for what could happen next. Rather than be emotional about the state of Jim, I deliberately willed myself to ignore emotions and focus on his medical condition, examining the facts.

When I decided it would be necessary to remove the first surgeon and replace him with Dr. Miller, I wanted to express myself in a way that would motivate the hospital administration to action. Without their action, Jim would not make it. Words can be powerful when used properly and thankfully, my email resulted in action. When I met the Chief Medical Officer, Dr. Paul

Douthitt, I remember looking him in the eye and smiling at him in hopes that he would like me! Being gracious and kind in critical situations is high gear!

The other thing to keep in mind is that to you--the patient or family member--this is a horrendous, life altering event. To them, it's clinical and they see life and death everyday--especially in ICU (Note to hospitals: Some ICU doctors are too used to death to be helpful and some have terrible bedside manner and communication skills. I think ICU doctors need training for this). *So what may seem unreal to you, the patient, may seem like another day at work to them.* I don't believe the team at Methodist views care in this way, but I'm sure many do. I say this not to discredit a medical team but to point out that they viewed my situation differently than I did. We both had the same objective to help Jim, but a family member needs to try and understand their perspective as well. It is also the medical team's responsibility to understand the patient's perspective. Some physicians are better than others and you must choose a physician according to your expectations.

Another thing about dealing with the medical profession is that you are going to get what you get if you stay in the hospital long enough, and some of it is not always pleasant. Largely, we had a great team and many of the nurses on 4-West became like family to us we were there so long. However, in any hospital, there will be difficult staff members who do not carry the cultural torch. We had a few. When this happens, you must try and avoid confrontation and stress. I often ignored those nurses who had a bad attitude or were rude. On a few occasions I did speak with someone higher up about it. But that was limited. The last thing you want to be is the "problem patient" on the floor. You must pick your battles and not sweat the small stuff. If you hang around a hospital long enough, you'll hear about it. I witnessed difficult and demanding patients on our floor who had unrealistic expectations and put stress and pressure on the medical staff. Do you think anyone wants to take care of a demanding, difficult, high-maintenance patient? No. High gear patients are those who respect the team and who know how to get along with others. Jim Howell is a patient in high gear. He kept a sense of humor and was quick to ask the nurses about their families. He rarely complained--even when in pain--and even joked about his bedsore he had. Many mornings when I arrived to Jim's room, he was in his chair trying his best to flirt and talk with sometimes two or three nurses. Even in pain and at his weakest, Jim was always gracious to everyone. I would think "wow, if he can do it, so can I."

## Jim Howell's Advice: How to be a high gear patient

"There is much of this experience that I thankfully don't remember. I think it was three weeks before I even knew what had happened to me. I was on so many pain meds and in the hospital for so long that much of the journey is a blur. Here is my advice if you are ever in the hospital for any duration of time:

- Treat your medical staff--especially the RNs with a great deal of respect
- Ask the nurses questions about their families so that they see you as a person, not just a patient
- If you are having a problem, tell your advocate and let them handle it
- If you are on a liquid diet for a month or more, seek expert help on foods you can prepare outside of the hospital such as soups, juices, etc that are healing
- Try to get PT to commit to a regular schedule
- Don't be afraid to have an advocate or RN to post a "no visitors" sign and coordinate visits with your advocate
- It's ok to cry--even for former rugby players
- If you are in for a long stay, don't be bashful about asking your doctor about taking a mild antidepressant which can also help you sleep better
- Make sure you are getting sunlight into your room if you can because you get days and nights mixed up. Patients need natural sunlight for healing and for emotional well being
- Take advantage of any excursion offered to leave your room like a wheel chair ride outside with a medical representative
- Have your advocate bring you loose fitting clothes and pajamas so that you are not confined to the hospital gown all the time. If you are getting up and able to walk around, bring your own shoes.
- Tell your advocate if you feel suicidal. It doesn't mean you will act on it, it is just normal to feel like you want to die when you have come so close several times.

- Finally, never agree to surgery by anyone until you have checked multiple references and friends in the medical community."

The important thing is to focus on healing and wellness and it takes a team to do this. If you are the advocate and spouse (like me) you have to think like a "team leader" and often I was the quarterback of Jim's status. I compared notes, asked questions, and adopted a proactive attitude to help Jim and the medical team. I like to solve problems, and tried hard to respect the team but would add my input when I thought it could be helpful. It's not what you say often, but how you say it. I was also there all of the time and I could be helpful eyes and ears to the medical team. I was watching Jim like a hawk most of the time. Hospitals are short staffed and I knew my presence there would be helpful, and it was.

Another important thing when dealing with the medical team is to understand their schedule and be there when they are doing rounds. After dropping Abby at school, I would race to get to the hospital in time for the 7:30-8:00 a.m. rounds. That was when I saw all the doctors and specialists and when the plan for the day was mapped out. Patient advocacy means being present and hearing everything the patient does. Often, as in our case, Jim could not hear or understand what decisions were being made so I had to be there and help the team coordinate these decisions for Jim.

## Surgeons

Just like anyone else, not all surgeons are created equal. This is a special breed of physician and one you hope you don't need but when you do, you had best do your due diligence to find the best at whatever it is you need done. Add to this that surgical errors are still high (too high) and below is a link supporting recent documentation.

The *Wall Street Journal* reported last year on the increase in surgical errors and high cost attributed to them (WSJ, *"How to Make Surgeries Safer: What Hospitals are doing to reduce human error"* by Laura Landro, published 2/16/15).

**YOU MUST:**

--Select the right surgeon the first time: ask questions, ask medical team members, ask nurses and make sure the surgeon you select has the skill and experience for the job. Meet with the surgeon prior to surgery and go over expectations to ensure you--the patient--understand the objectives.

--Removing a bad surgeon from a case: As it became obvious to us that the first surgeon was not responsive and non-communicative, I decided to seek the hospital's help (as described previously). You must be firm and stick to facts. When the first surgeon wanted to speak to me as he was being moved off the case, I held my ground and told him I had no confidence in him and that I didn't want him on the case. I didn't cry, yell, cuss or punch him (like I felt like doing). I looked him straight in the eye and told him directly how it was going to be.

--Meeting the new surgeon for Jim's case: I have already said that Dr. Mark Miller is a fantastic person and surgeon. We know this now but did not know then. As he took the case and became immediately immersed doing emergency surgery to save Jim, I established that he and I would work well together because he is a **good communicator.** He gave me his cell and told me to text him with anything I needed. My job was to make sure I didn't blow up his phone and I would save questions and write them down so that I could ask them all at one time. So learning how to best communicate with your medical team is a key strategy. Some prefer to call you after hours. Some prefer texts. Ask your medical team how they like to communicate and assure them you will not abuse it.

In Jim's case, there was so much going on that Dr. Miller would ask me to text him photos of Jim's wound, etc. as we changed dressings. That way, he could see what it looked like if he couldn't be there when wound care arrived. Simple strategies like that contribute to the overall care of the patient. And a good surgeon will appreciate a curious advocate because it helps him (or her) do a better job.

--Surgeons are usually the ones who lead the team and Dr. Miller certainly was in our case. All the other specialists will coordinate and confer with the surgeon. It is even more important---when things get complex--to have someone who works well with others. While many do, we learned the hard way, that some do not.

## Hospital Administration

We were (and still are) fortunate that Jim had his surgery--even the first one--at Methodist Le Bonheur Hospital Germantown. I think we'd be hard pressed to find a better system and for the Methodist team, we are grateful. Hospital administrators--really great ones--are worth their weight in gold when it comes to problem solving. I have already stated how I worked closely with them to help Jim, but here are some high gear tips--from my experience--for dealing with the administration:

--Go directly to the top in a crisis and let the CEO know what is taking place and do it by an email. If you don't know the CEO, find out who he/she is and get to know them
--Use facts and document your reason(s) for problems, changes
--Do not threaten anyone in administration with calling media, filing a lawsuit, etc. I actually witnessed a conversation between a patient and a medical team member where the patient was yelling she would call Channel 5
--Put yourself in their shoes if you can and remember, they see it everyday
--Be polite to everyone and get to know the administrative team in the hospital. Several times I stopped in to say hello to the kind women working at the front desk in administration. When we were stuck for days in the hospital and Abby had mandatory community service hours to achieve for school, these ladies gave her some! We didn't even have to leave the hospital for Abby to get in her community service hours
--View the administration as your advocate not the enemy. I think people have a negative perception that a hospital is a big, money-hungry machine and that they don't care as long as they get paid. This is not the

case, and while it is important for hospitals to be profitable, it is more important to most to provide the best quality care. If you have a question or a problem during a hospital stay and you cannot get a solution from a clinician or social worker, turn to someone in administration for guidance

## Here are some wise words from Mr. William Kenley, CEO of Methodist Le Bonheur Germantown Hospital:

*"Patients and families come to us for help. Hospitals must have policies, procedures, and processes to ensure we provide the very best, evidence-based clinical care. Much is written about the need to drive out inconsistency in healthcare delivery and reduce opportunity for error. While our organization is sharply focused on these opportunities, we also understand that policies and procedures cannot substitute for highly trained, caring professionals who exercise their skill and compassion to connect with our patients and families and provide them our very best.*

*Jim's story points out how a healthcare team works at its very best. It is interesting to note that this excellence is founded on very basic principles. First, make a connection between the patient and family and the clinicians providing care. Second, listen to understand their needs. And finally, honor commitments and follow through. Amy shares examples of both failed and successful communication. While she certainly loved hearing "good news", it was obvious that the more basic need was to hear the truth.*

*Patient and family engagement are key to having the best healthcare experience. Engaged patients have a more fulfilling and better experience. Jim points out some great points to consider when we find ourselves as "the patient". I am proud of our team here at Methodist Le Bonheur Germantown Hospital. We have a special and strong culture. We are not perfect, but that is our goal. Working together with families like the Howells is a privilege for us. Their engagement and feedback helps us accelerate our journey toward providing excellence to every patient and family we serve, every single day and every single time."*

## Medical Teams (PA's, RN's, OT's, Wound Care, PT, Aides, Social Workers, Home health, etc)

In a hospital, you only see your doctor(s) periodically depending on your case. Who you do see everyday are the teams assigned to your case and they work in 12-hour shifts. Their schedules float and it is common to have a variety of people on your case. At Methodist, they strive for continuity of care so with Jim, the RNs on 4-West became familiar with Jim's case. We often had repeat staff on his case. It helps when the medical team is familiar with the issues, especially when they were as complex as they were for us.

These people are the ones you will interact with daily and frequently. They perform a variety of duties and I learned hardly ever get a break. If the hospital or floor is busy, they will be pulled in numerous directions. These are the people you need on your team. You need them to like you, and you need to be very nice to them. It is easy to forget in clinical settings that people are still people first. It was important to me for the staff to like Jim and my family if we were going to get him well. An important note as well is that some of the nurses had great ideas and input that I was able to later ask the doctors about. These are the people that are with the patients the most and a good team will value their input. In a long-term medical situation like ours, I also knew it was important to have a positive experience as possible.

## High gear tips for engaging with medical teams

--Don't hover over their station if you need something. Just stand out by your door and they will ask you

--Be aware that you are not the only patient and they have busy jobs. Sometimes we forget because it is human nature to focus on ourselves. Think of the other patients on the floor and be aware of how full the floor is. I could always tell when it would be busy and when it wouldn't and could adjust to help Jim accordingly

--Bring the staff food and flowers. I fed ICU at least 6 times and 4-West more than that. Eating is often what the staff can't do so bringing food to them is helpful and gracious and especially when the weather is nasty and parking is an issue. The more the staff likes you, the better for everyone

--Offer to help. I emptied urinals, bathed Jim, helped him up, fed him, helped him brush his teeth, and other duties to help out

--Be your patient's eyes and ears. If you are advocating for a patient and you think something is wrong, you need to say something. It's better to over communicate than to under communicate

--Document things so when you have a shift change--even though it's in the charts--you can help reinforce the patient status

# CHAPTER 7

## A word--or several--about Insurance Companies

"I have never had a client who said that their
spouse purchased too much insurance"
--Jack Dewald, Agency Services Inc.

### The Current Status of most Health Insurance Plans

Choice is a foundational principle in a well-functioning capitalist marketplace. In the healthcare space patient choice has been hijacked by large payer systems and networks. Gone are the days when a patient may independently decide who provides their medical care. That decision now primarily rests with the patient's health plan – a plan that was likely chosen by an employer or the government, but not the patient.

This health plan selects the panel of doctors, the hospitals, the surgery centers, the laboratories and all ancillary services that may be needed by their covered population. The plan also interjects itself into the medical decisions made by its panel of providers sometimes contradicting that provider's best advice. This system has been adopted in order to decrease the cost of medical care, but a higher cost has been incurred by the patient who no longer has the freedom to make the extremely personal choice of who treats their medical condition.

While it is true that some profiteering providers have abused the system by ordering more tests than necessary let's consider how those same profiteers will address the new model of setting fixed prices with fixed provider panels.

In the new world these folks will provide fewer procedures, including necessary procedures, in order to increase the margin between revenue and cost. Their highest profit will occur when they perform fewer procedures. It won't take long for their patients to suffer, but money will be saved!

The better approach is to return to the patient the ability to choose the provider of this intimate care and to be responsible for choosing wisely. Patients should not be restricted to a panel of providers and facilities chosen for them by a bureaucratic system. In our information-rich society patients are increasingly able to make well informed decisions regarding healthcare, indeed health plans expect patients to be better informed--even to bear more of the cost through higher deductibles and co-payments. With higher costs you might expect more patient choice, but just the opposite has happened.

In my opinion, insurance plans should be required to offer open access to any provider willing to accept their rates of reimbursement. Patients should be able to select from all willing providers. Several more issues would need to be addressed in order to create a better functioning healthcare market, but the dynamic of patient choice is foundational to every other issue.

Personally, our insurance premiums have gone up by 60% and are now more than our house note. You know the saying "the rich get richer and the poor get poorer," well it's headed there if not already. While not all insurance monopolies are corrupt, I think universal reform is critical to the future of our healthcare delivery system.

## Why You Need Insurance

Thankfully, Jim and I had planned long ago for buying life and disability insurance although we have not used either. We also have always had health insurance and would have been in bankruptcy if we had not had it when this happened. Both Jim and I are fortunate in that we have always worked around CPAs, lawyers, estate planners and insurance brokers. I have known for a long time the role insurance can have on a family and now that I have seen it first hand, I think it is an important part of a family's ability to survive a medical crisis.

Jack Dewald is a client (ASI in Memphis) and good friend who has worked in the life, health and disability insurance business for many years. He came to see me often at the hospital and helped me with some of our insurance options and considerations. In anticipation of the possibility (at the time, probability) of Jim not making it, I asked Jack to review our insurance policies and give me some advice. He did and I also wanted him to contribute here in this chapter. Here is some good information from Jack as it relates to our story:

## Jack Dewald, CLU, RHU of Agency Services Inc. (ASI Memphis)

"People brag about a new car or new jewelry the bought but in my experience over 35 years in the insurance industry, nobody brags about what a great insurance package they have. In fact, most people never talk about it until that big claim comes around and then they are REALLY glad they have that insurance. As one of Amy's clients, I saw first hand the many impacts Jim's surgery and complications caused for the Howell family. Insurance played a big role in their situation. First of all, they have **medical insurance.** Sure everybody hates paying premiums but when a major hospitalization occurs, the bills easily reach into the hundreds of thousands of dollars. In Jim's case, he had good major medical insurance that paid the majority of his bills. Although his deductible is high, without this coverage, the Howells would be bankrupt.

The Howells also have **disability insurance** which--unfortunately--they cannot claim until a certain timeframe has elapsed. If they do opt for it later, it can help replace income they have lost due to this illness and the inability to work. They also have **life insurance** which thankfully they did not need. Amy spoke candidly about several close calls where Jim's medical team were not certain he would live. That's scary stuff. Nobody ever wants to talk about dying, but part of the planning includes planning to die well. This includes making plans for your family long after you are gone. We buy life insurance because we love our families. When someone who dies has purchased life insurance, it means their kids get to stay in the same private school and their spouse gets to stay in their home. It replaces lost income and allows a family to live in dignity. Jim's life insurance gave Amy the peace of mind that if the worse happened she would be financially prepared to deal with it.

Too often people think insurance is for older people and when young, people think something cannot happen. Very wrong. We see spouses pass suddenly-for various reasons-and we are always glad to be able to deliver the big benefit. I've never had a widow tell me their spouse bought too much life insurance. Thankfully, Amy and Jim's wise planning and execution of purchasing insurance has them in the position they are in. Often, when something as tragic as this happens, past a certain age, you may be ineligible to purchase life insurance. Don't wait until you cannot get it to get it."

Thank you Jack Dewald! For more great information, you can visit the Agency Services Inc. website at www.agencyservices.com and follow Jack on Twitter @JackDewald and read his blog. Jack is also the author of a book, "Ten Sales Concepts to Relish Remember & Repeat"--a guide to how life insurance provides security for loved ones. You may order the book by emailing Jack at JDewald@AgencyServices.com. If you can't reach Jack because he's duck hunting in Arkansas, you can call and ask for Angie Pettinger (COO) or Rena King (Rockstar Rena).

## Summing it all Up

This chapter highlights the macro level industry wide, national health insurance issues that are problematic when it comes to patient access and care. The second part of the chapter highlights why we need insurance. We must work nationally to improve the industry, allow better access and more patient controlled choices while still being able to have health insurance that works best for the individual patient. It is not an easy dilemma and probably won't be "fixed" in my lifetime unfortunately.

# CHAPTER 8

## How to Survive 90+ days in a Hospital

"Give us this day our daily bread"
--THE LORD'S PRAYER

Nothing can prepare you for a trauma or tragedy that seems to last forever--especially when you don't see it coming. Our experience has taught us that life is precious, fleeting and you must focus on one day at a time. People have always said this, but once you have something so traumatic happen, you really understand it and appreciate it. Our lives are normally so busy with our careers, families, children, sports, church, etc., that we hardly stop and think about living for today. I think this is the biggest lesson of all that we have learned and in a strange way, it is a gift. The ability to truly be grateful and mindful of each day has given me a deeper faith, a clearer path and--although change abounds--has changed me for the better. I think that which doesn't kill you makes you stronger and so we are stronger for what we have been through. I don't recommend it voluntarily though!

Our children rallied around us, as did their friends and did not give us one ounce of drama during this past year. We are proud of them and believe they truly "stepped up" in big ways. My hope is that they will never have to go through anything like it again, but if they do, they will know how to handle it.

One of the hardest things ever is to have to be in a hospital for a long period of time. It's emotionally draining, it's physically challenging, it's unpleasant at times, it's limiting and it can be downright depressing. At one point during our journey, when I thought Jim would not make it out, I believe I was truly depressed. I was at the end of my rope, as it had already been several months of in and out of ICU. It is easy to get depressed when you are the one taking care of everything and seeing your spouse deteriorating. And I'm not weaker for expressing how I felt, I just think honesty is important. And I add here how much the Methodist administration knew this, helped me and was patient with me sometimes when I was at my wit's end. I recall fondly sweet Donna Abney calling my cell to check on me and she caught the brunt of some serious frustrations from me that day! Thankfully, Donna is a high gear woman and we were in the class of 1993 (the best class) Leadership Memphis together. I pretty much vented and probably cussed about a few things but Donna just listened and helped me. Kudos to the team at Methodist.

Adding to feelings of frustration and depression was the thought of Jim's physical condition. Yes, it could be worse, but Jim was in a pretty awful state for awhile. This is not easy on any spouse. My whole life--as I knew it--had been flipped upside down. I deserved to be depressed at times, but a little voice inside me would say "Amy, stop it." I found that I had to keep moving forward and try and do for others where I could. Helping other people is a great way to divert your attention elsewhere. So I worked when I could, focusing on clients when they needed me, and I brought food to the hospital for the staff. These actions were my "coping mechanisms."

I should also insert here that my co-author of my two books (_Women in High Gear_ and _The Future Belongs to Students in High Gear_) and I were working on book number two and all during Jim's hospital stay, I could work some on writing the book. We published this guide for students as they go from class to career in September of 2015. Both books are now on Amazon and when all of this happened to Jim, I told my co-author and great friend, Anne D. Gallaher that I had to write "Healing in High Gear." Writing for me is a great diversion and I think it's important to use your experiences to help other people. What good is all of the knowledge if we don't share it, right?

## High gear tips for getting through staying in a hospital for an extended period of time

--Pray everyday and often: When something bad happens like it did to us, only God knows what will happen. Prayer is the best path to help heal and also a great coping mechanism for trauma. I would start my day with prayer and end it with prayer. If you are praying, you aren't worrying (as much) and if you are worrying you aren't praying. Now, whenever I worry about something, I pray about it instead

--Wear comfortable clothes and shoes always

--Bring your own pillows to the hospital for you and the patient with fresh cases

--Bring a foam "topper" and sheets for the cot or sofa you have to sleep on--it helps

--Eat healthy when you can and exercise when you can. I did more healthy eating than I did exercise but I did my best. You have to give yourself a break and not be hard on yourself when you are going through this. That can be difficult for more "type A" people like I have a tendency to be. What I learned is you just have to do what is right each day for your patient and family. That often means you cannot workout as much and that's ok as long as you move and walk. I would walk the hospital floors and go out to my car just to stretch my legs and get a break

--Don't eat the hospital food--get out and get in a non-clinical place for breaks

--Establish a communication system for visitors. One thing I learned is that people like to stop by the hospital unannounced. This can be confusing if you have left to run an errand or if the patient is gone in the CT lab. **If you are going to visit someone, please be courteous and at least text them that you want to come.** In Jim's case there were times when he could have no visitors and I would meet people in the waiting area. I think establishing updates on a social site like Facebook is a good way to inform a lot of people and maintain some privacy and space

--When you know you shouldn't let the patient have visitors, get the RNs to post a sign on the door. We posted "NO Visitors" on Jim's door several times throughout his journey for a number of reasons. Don't be afraid to tell people no and that it's not convenient to drop by. And one tip:

**night time is generally not the best time to visit patients**. Their days start early--often they are up multiple times during the night--and by evening, they are tired. Everyone is--Visit but keep it short
--Open the shades during the day so patients know it's daytime
--Decorate the hospital room if you can! Jim's room was at least cheery and we had fun putting up inspirational messages and notes on his wall
--Keep a journal daily. Writing for me is calming and liberating. In the thick of things, it helped me to keep a daily log of everything from what the doctors said to the meds Jim was on to how many liters of urine he expelled, etc. Once you record it, you can free up your mind and refer to it later if needed. And in Jim's case, he missed most of what happened as he was either sedated, in ICU or on pain meds. A journal lets the patient read later what happened
--Keep a cooler in the hospital room with foods you love
--Take vitamins and drink juices made from shops like the Juice Bar (Scott Tashie)
--Know when you need to be there and when you don't. In our case, initially I was there almost around the clock. As time went on, I knew when I could leave for a bit and when I needed to be there. When you can get out and get breaks, do it
--Pamper yourself IF you can. I think spas and massages inside hospitals would be a great revenue producer and an amenity I needed! They have them in airports now, so they could also have them in hospitals

Note to hospital facility management people: Can we get more daylight and natural light in the hospitals? Can we have food courts and juice bars in common areas that serve healthy options? Can we have a nail shop, massage therapy and other "for pay" retail in hospitals for people who desperately need those services but cannot leave the hospital (not patients but families of patients)? These services would be value adds for hospitals and ancillary revenue producers.

# CHAPTER 9

## Balancing running a Business and your Family while your Spouse is in the Hospital

"Either you run the day....or the day runs you"
--ANONYMOUS

'm not going to sugar coat it. Taking care of an ill spouse can be more than a full-time job. If I had not had a good team in place who could support me, I would have lost my business completely. Thankfully, I had experienced help in my shop during the stormiest parts of our journey.

When it all started, the first thing I did was notify all of my clients--many of whom are friends and many came to visit. They only emailed me when they really needed me--and some did--and I kept my laptop handy everyday so as to not miss anything critical. I leaned on my team and let them handle much of the load. They did a fantastic job and I will be forever grateful. Specifically I am grateful to Lacey Washburn, Sarah Womack, Marc Burford, Glen Gilmore and to my co-author and friend, Anne Deeter Gallaher. These wonderful people all contributed to me keeping things moving and supporting me in some ways. I am also grateful to Alys Drake, Audrey Evensky Brantz and Molly Evensky Bernatsky who were always standing by to help with any special work related projects. The reality is that I was able to spend so much time taking care of Jim and focusing on his health.

It wasn't easy however. A few times I had to tear myself away from the hospital and go to a meeting. Even when Jim was on his deathbed I had a client that demanded I be present in a meeting. Understandably, as business is business. However, this journey has made me re-think what I do and how I do it in my firm. I believe it has prepared me for the next chapter in my business. Specifically, it has taught me that life is too short for negative people and clients who want everything but don't want to pay for it. Time is the one thing we cannot get more of, so why waste it?

I don't know how I balanced everything and sometimes I didn't so such a great job. At times I felt like I was doing it all halfway but when something like this happens, you do the best you can and start over the next day. As I have said, one blessing was that our kids didn't need much parenting. They needed my time and love and I gave that to them. We had to skip sporting events, movies, family dinners and things families normally do. My kids had to be self-sufficient, visit the hospital, get homework done and rely on each other to help them get what they needed and get to school. I remember thinking often how fortunate we were to have Abby at St. Benedict at Auburndale--a loving, caring school that supported us and especially Abby. When something happens, it happens to the whole family--not just the patient.

Think about when you really feel you have balance. It is surely not going to be during trauma. So the point here is that I managed it but there were days when I was off balance and out of balance. There were days when I did not get out of my pj's or shower. There were days I almost didn't recognize the face looking back at me in the mirror.

Recovering from such a nightmare is what is critical. If you fall down seven times, you get up eight. You have to get through it the best way you can and then get over and beyond it. As I write this, this is almost where I am. We still have Jim's last and hopefully final surgery coming. We are not quite yet fully recovered but we are moving in the right direction.

## High gear tips for keeping your work/business going

--get help if you can: reallocate work and plan for what's coming
--notify your clients/customers of the situation: most will stay with you

--do what you can remotely during breaks: working can be therapeutic for you

--hire extra hands if needed

--try to do 1 really great thing for a client each week

--get your banker and cpa involved even if it means paying extra

--if you have a line of credit, you will need it

--thank your team and keep them informed of all updates

--forgive yourself if you lose business or revenue--it's part of it

--apply your new experiences to your business (I'm writing this book for example)

--remember that you will get out of this and be back someday: don't lose faith

# CHAPTER 10

## Hospitals: Transparency and Accountability

> "Given all of the current technology, strategies and tools that
> are available to prevent these occurrences, it is unacceptable
> that foreign objects are still being left in surgical sites
> and that wrong-site surgeries are still occurring, "
> -- LISA FREEMAN, EXECUTIVE DIRECTOR OF THE NONPROFIT

Connecticut Center for Patient Safety.

On June 22 of 2015, the "Health Affairs Blog" published a post by Robert Watcher entitled "You Can't Understand Something you Hide: Transparency As A Path To Improve Patient Safety.' In this article is a true story about a woman who died as a result of a simple medical error--filling a syringe with the wrong substance and injecting into the woman. The story went on to say that the clinical team took full responsibility for the error, owned up to what happened and even revealed the error to the entire staff, highlighting a problem and promising to improve from it.

On February 16, 2015, the *Wall Street Journal* (WSJ) reported on "How to Make Surgery Safer--Going under the knife is riskier than it should be. What hospitals are doing to reduce human error."

The article says that in an analysis done in 2014 in the journal Patient Safety in Surgery, 46% to 65% of adverse events in hospitals are related to surgery, particularly the complex surgeries. According to the article, hospitals are using data to track performance and adhere to best practices. They are also trying to educate surgeons about using potentially dangerous equipment as well as paying attention to team members and safety in the operating room.

"Given all of the current technology, strategies and tools that are available to prevent these occurrences, it is unacceptable that foreign objects are still being left in surgical sites and that wrong-site surgeries are still occurring, " said Lisa Freeman, executive director of the nonprofit Connecticut Center for Patient Safety--quoted in the WSJ story.

The article goes on to report the tremendous costs of these errors and what some are doing about it. Like the other post, you cannot improve a hospital's surgical quality if you can't see and measure it.

According to the WSJ, Johns Hopkins, Surgery; Centers for Disease Control and Prevention released these U.S. figures:

39: The number of times a week a surgeon leaves a foreign object such as a sponge or a towel inside a patient's body after an operation.

20: The number of times a week a surgeon performs the wrong procedure on a patient.

20: The number of times a week a surgeon operates on the wrong site.

157,000: The number of surgical-site infections in 2013
http://www/wsj/com/articles/how-to-make-surgery-safer-1424145652

There are numerous studies out there about safety but I believe safety is the first step toward transparency. Hospitals who cannot admit mistakes and correct them will likely not be able to compete in the future. Also important is a surgeon who will be a team player and work well with the operating room to ensure safety.

After going through this journey, I believe that Methodist Le Bonheur Healthcare has set the bar high for both safety and transparency. While there is always room for improvement--in any system--I know Methodist strives for the best outcomes. With the exception of the first surgery (which was directly attributed to the first surgeon himself) we had--overall--a very open relationship with the medical team and administration. Methodist has clearly instilled a culture of transparent care in a faith-based community.

# CHAPTER 11

## Purpose of this book and How
## Helping Others Helps You

> "One must really have suffered oneself to help others,"
> --Mother Teresa

f you have read this far, by now you are getting the picture that I am writing this because it is therapeutic and a way for me to give back and also to help others who are in similar situations or maybe will be someday. I have always found that one way to get yourself out of a blue mood is to do something good for someone else. Helping others feels good and can be very healing for you. Additionally, if this book can help a spouse or advocate save a life, then it is so worth it.

I have had a lot of people say, "Amy, I don't know how you did it," or "Amy, I don't think I would know what to do like you did," or "Amy, if something happens to me I want you there." All common things people are saying to me now. I even have one friend who has me in her phone as her emergency contact.

I hope this book can be and will be helpful to many for a long time to come. One thing I will share here is that if you bought this book, a portion of the proceeds will be going to the the hospital's foundation which exists to help others. I imagine if this book is a great seller, we'll be able to do some good work for sepsis awareness and patient advocacy to help a lot of people who need it.

My belief is that when something so tragic and terrible happens as it did to us, we must make something good come out of it. I want to use this book as my calling card to help others. My hope is that I can tell our story to others and shed light on the issues talked about here in this book. I want "Healing in High Gear" to be a common theme known across hospital systems for helping not only patients but their families and caregivers especially. I want a single mom with two small kids who has an accident to know that resources are out there to help her family. That is the purpose and soul of this evergreen book.

# CHAPTER 12

## Healing Scripture Verses

The following Bible verses from both Old and New Testament are great and uplifting to read when you have a minute or two and even want to share them. I thought I'd put them in here because during one of our ICU visits a volunteer from the hospital gave me a small slip of paper with a Bible verse on it and I thought how kind it was and read it several times, and it helped me so much. I also left some white spaces here to encourage you to write in some of your own thoughts here on these pages if you feel so moved.

I believe God does have a plan and He does hear our prayers. If you are reading this while in the hospital, I hope these scripture passages can provide comfort and help you along your journey.

**Acts 5:16**
16 The people also gathered from the towns around Jerusalem, bringing the sick and those afflicted with unclean spirits, and they were all healed.

**Romans 8:11**
11 If the Spirit of him who raised Jesus from the dead dwells in you, he who raised Christ Jesus from the dead will also give life to your mortal bodies through his Spirit who dwells in you.

**2 Corinthians 4:10-11**
10 always carrying in the body the death of Jesus, so that the life of Jesus may also be manifested in our bodies. 11 For we who live are

always being given over to death for Jesus' sake, so that the life of Jesus also may be manifested in our mortal flesh.

### Deuteronomy 11:21
21 that your days and the days of your children may be multiplied in the land that the Lord swore to your fathers to give them, as long as the heavens are above the earth.

### Deuteronomy 7:15
15 And the Lord will take away from you all sickness, and none of the evil diseases of Egypt, which you knew, will he inflict on you, but he will lay them on all who hate you.

### Mark 16:17-18
17 And these signs will accompany those who believe: in my name they will cast out demons; they will speak in new tongues; 18 they will pick up serpents with their hands; and if they drink any deadly poison, it will not hurt them; they will lay their hands on the sick, and they will recover."

### Isaiah 40:31
31 but they who wait for the Lord shall renew their strength;
they shall mount up with wings like eagles;
they shall run and not be weary;
they shall walk and not faint.

### Psalm 34:19
19 Many are the afflictions of the righteous,
but the Lord delivers him out of them all.

### Jeremiah 30:17
17 For I will restore health to you,
and your wounds I will heal,
declares the Lord,
because they have called you an outcast:
'It is Zion, for whom no one cares!'

### Isaiah 53:4-5

4 Surely he has borne our griefs
and carried our sorrows;
yet we esteemed him stricken,
smitten by God, and afflicted.
5 But he was wounded for our transgressions;
he was crushed for our iniquities;
upon him was the chastisement that brought us peace,
and with his stripes we are healed.

### Jeremiah 33:6

6 Behold, I will bring to it health and healing, and I will heal them
and reveal to them abundance of prosperity and security.

### Mark 11:24

24 Therefore I tell you, whatever you ask in prayer, believe that you
have received it, and it will be yours.

### Isaiah 58:8

8 Then shall your light break forth like the dawn,
and your healing shall spring up speedily;
your righteousness shall go before you;
the glory of the Lord shall be your rear guard.

### Psalm 41:3

3 The Lord sustains him on his sickbed;
in his illness you restore him to full health.

### Romans 8:32

32 He who did not spare his own Son but gave him up for us all, how
will he not also with him graciously give us all things?

### Psalm 34:10

10 The young lions suffer want and hunger;
but those who seek the Lord lack no good thing.

**Psalm 103:3**
3 who forgives all your iniquity,
who heals all your diseases,

**Isaiah 53:5**
5 But he was wounded for our transgressions;
he was crushed for our iniquities;
upon him was the chastisement that brought us peace,
and with his stripes we are healed.

**Psalm 119:93**
93 I will never forget your precepts,
for by them you have given me life.

**John 8:36**
36 So if the Son sets you free, you will be free indeed.

**Romans 8:2**
2 For the law of the Spirit of life has set you free in Christ Jesus from
the law of sin and death.

**John 1:2**
2 Beloved, I pray that all may go well with you and that you may be
in good health, as it goes well with your soul.

**1 Peter 2:24**
24 He himself bore our sins in his body on the tree, that we might die
to sin and live to righteousness. By his wounds you have been healed.

**Isaiah 40:29**
29 He gives power to the faint,
and to him who has no might he increases strength.

**Jeremiah 30:17**
17 For I will restore health to you,

and your wounds I will heal,
declares the Lord,
because they have called you an outcast

**Matthew 8:17**
17 This was to fulfill what was spoken by the prophet Isaiah: "He took our illnesses and bore our diseases."

**Isaiah 40:31**
31 but they who wait for the Lord shall renew their strength;
they shall mount up with wings like eagles;
they shall run and not be weary;
they shall walk and not faint.

**Romans 8:11**
11 If the Spirit of him who raised Jesus from the dead dwells in you, he who raised Christ Jesus from the dead will also give life to your mortal bodies through his Spirit who dwells in you.

**Proverbs 3:7-8**
7 Be not wise in your own eyes;
fear the Lord, and turn away from evil.
8 It will be healing to your flesh
and refreshment to your bones.

**Proverbs 4:20-22**
20 My son, be attentive to my words;
incline your ear to my sayings.
21 Let them not escape from your sight;
keep them within your heart.
22 For they are life to those who find them,
and healing to all their flesh.

**Psalm 42:11**
11 Why are you cast down, O my soul,
and why are you in turmoil within me?

Hope in God; for I shall again praise him,
my salvation and my God.

**Psalm 107:20**
20 He sent out his word and healed them,
and delivered them from their destruction.

**Jeremiah 33:6**
6 Behold, I will bring to it health and healing, and I will heal them
and reveal to them abundance of prosperity and security.

**Psalm 46:1**
46:1 God is our refuge and strength,
a very present help in trouble.

**Psalm 55:22**
22 Cast your burden on the Lord,
and he will sustain you;
he will never permit
the righteous to be moved.

**Psalm 25:20**
20 Oh, guard my soul, and deliver me!
Let me not be put to shame, for I take refuge in you.

**Jeremiah 17:14**
14 Heal me, O Lord, and I shall be healed;
save me, and I shall be saved,
for you are my praise.

**Psalm 119:107**
107 I am severely afflicted;
give me life, O Lord, according to your word!

**Psalm 121:2**
2 My help comes from the Lord,

who made heaven and earth.

**Psalm 119:50**
50 This is my comfort in my affliction,
that your promise gives me life.

**Psalm 116:10**
10 I believed, even when I spoke,
"I am greatly afflicted";

**Isaiah 43:2**
2 When you pass through the waters, I will be with you;
and through the rivers, they shall not overwhelm you;
when you walk through fire you shall not be burned,
and the flame shall not consume you.

**Exodus 15:26**
26 saying, "If you will diligently listen to the voice of the Lord
your God, and do that which is right in his eyes, and give ear to
his commandments and keep all his statutes, I will put none of
the diseases on you that I put on the Egyptians, for I am the Lord,
your healer."

**Deuteronomy 7:15**
15 And the Lord will take away from you all sickness, and none of the
evil diseases of Egypt, which you knew, will he inflict on you, but he
will lay them on all who hate you.

**Deuteronomy 7:14**
14 You shall be blessed above all peoples. There shall not be male or
female barren among you or among your livestock.

**James 5:16**

16 Therefore, confess your sins to one another and pray for one another, that you may be healed. The prayer of a righteous person has great power as it is working.

**Hebrews 13:8**

8 Jesus Christ is the same yesterday and today and forever.

# CHAPTER 13

## The Final Surgery: June 14, 2016

5:00 A.M.: The big, long-awaited day is finally here! We set our alarms to get up at 4:00 A.M. and Jim showered and dressed to go. Thankful that McDonald's has a 24-hour drive through, I grabbed a small coffee. Poor Jim has to drink some type of "prep" drink and hasn't had any food since Sunday.

Arrived at Methodist LeBonheur Germantown Hospital as instructed, checked in, and got to surgery to do all of the pre-op work. Dr. Miller came in to see us and said, "we're going in to attach everything and we'll be there for awhile but I'll keep you updated."

7:00 A.M.: I just left Jim who is getting an epidural block in advance of general anesthesia and surgery will be underway shortly. I'm listening to Fox News in the surgery wait and glad I brought my Mac to finish this chapter. I expect to see Mona Sappenfiled and Alys Drake soon....during long surgeries, it is nice to have people to support you and help pass the time.

Mona brought coffee and cookies and Alys joined us as we sat in surgery waiting. Finally about 9:00 I got a call on my cell phone from Thomas, the OR RN who said the surgery started at about 8:40.

Around 11:00, Thomas called and said surgery still going well and that Dr. Miller had not yet reached the colon--so much scar tissue and complex, intricate work. With that call, we moved out to the hospital's main lobby for a change of scenery and to get away from a crowded, noisy surgery waiting area. Mona brought a massage therapist to the hospital to give us a chair massage and that was a great way to burn an hour! Alys went to get lunch and my parents showed up to wait with us as did Kelly Truitt.

Finally, about 1:45, Dr. Miller came to find us with a smile on his face! "It was tough but we did it. I got his colon re-attached, put new mesh in and did everything I could to make sure it's good and connected, " said Miller. He told us that the plastic surgeon, Dr. Robert Chandler would be finishing up and surgery would go a bit longer. They were putting staples and stitches down his abdominal cavity and closing him up! Later, around 2:45, Dr. Chandler came out to tell us Jim was going to be in recovery for a few hours and after that would go to ICU but would not be sedated or on the ventilator! Thank you God!

Jim spent two days in ICU just to be sure all was well and then went to room 428 on 4 West. It is almost Father's Day now and we've been in the hospital for five days. They have just removed Jim's epidural and pain management will now be as needed by mouth. The "ERAS" method of surgery is great. Apparently it is widely used in Europe (began in Denmark) and is a better way for invasive surgical recovery. Basically, the patient gets an epidural that slowly releases pain medication to the area of need--the abdomen--versus drugging the whole body and mind. ERAS stands for "Enhanced Recovery" and it has definitely been a great approach for Jim. Dr. Miller says "we don't have to beat you up so much to build you back up." It apparently speeds recovery and is better for everyone.

## Father's Day: June 19, 2016:

We are still in the hospital but expect to go home early next week where Jim will heal and continue to recover. Recovery time for him is approximately six to eight weeks. Dr. Miller wants everything to heal without complication. A full recovery means Jim will be back to normal without the ostomy bag, have a working colon and intestinal tract. He will not be able to do any "core workouts" or strenuous exercise for one year from now. Dr. Miller wants his abdominal cavity to heal for a year.

We will finally have our life back with an impressive set of scars to show for the trauma we endured. I'd say it's a pretty great Father's Day to be on the "other side" of this last surgery. Let us hope and pray that Jim continues to heal and gets far beyond this--without any permanent complications--to regain a full life again.

# Acknowledgements

To all of our "prayer warriors" out there, we credit you for helping save Jim's life.

I thank the congregations at Germantown Presbyterian Church, Government Street Presbyterian Church (Mobile, AL) as well as congregations across Memphis and the country. The best gift basket ever came from the Olive Branch Church of Christ and Lynn Stephens. The best gifts I got came from Kathy Snavely (superman cape) and Xan Pearson (prayer blanket)--my social media powerhouse friends who are also friends in real life. I am grateful for the chaplains at Methodist Le Bonheur Germantown, the ministers at GPC, Jay Howell and Will Jones especially who prayed with me and for us often.

To our great friends--so many to list but those who came to the hospital, brought us food, bought gift cards, donated time and money, you helped carry us through this ordeal and I am forever grateful. To my many family members from Texas and friends on Facebook--I love you and all of your supportive, loving comments which I read daily. I printed them all off for keepsake and will never forget how much that support meant to me--always will.

To my family, my parents, our children, Bryan and Abby--there are really no words to express my love and gratitude for you daily. You are all inspirational, loving and by definition, the best anyone could ask for. God blessed us with you two great kids. I am also grateful for your crew of friends who were with us often both at the hospital and our home. I love "all my children"-- Somer, Rachel, Jacob, Matthew, Callan, Connor, Pearce, Blake, Kinner, Matt, Cooke...thank you for your visits to the hospital. I know it wasn't easy and you cheer us up so much. Thank you for supporting Bryan and Abby!

To my sisters, Blythe and Heather--you rock. Love you to the moon and back. And Heather, I am especially glad you were there so much to rub my feet and back and make me laugh when I needed it. And the many mornings you brought me "coffee Dollface."

To my aunts, uncles and cousins on the Donaho side, I love you all and appreciate all that you have done. We need another "river reunion" when this is all over! To my mom's family on the Ferguson side, thank you for the prayers and support.

To Anne Gallaher, my co-author and great friend, thank you for helping me in so many ways get our second book finished and published. I love our collaboration together and also love our special reunions for good food and "guac" as we ate our way through Texas. We are grateful to Bob Akin who launched our book at TCU and to the wonderful Windegger family whom we love so much and have for so long! More great times ahead and we need more cowboy boots, right?

To Methodist Le Bonheur Germantown and the entire medical team-- Jim would not be here without you. Special thanks to Shannon, Dr. Susan Murrmann, Dr. Martin Weiss and the absolute star of the show: Dr. Mark Miller. I would not have had him if it hadn't been for Dr. Murrmann's great assist and the hospital administration's (William Kenley and Dr. Paul Douthitt) fast action. We are eternally grateful.

To the absolutely most incredible caregivers, the RN's at Methodist: We realize the amazing work you all do everyday with a smile on your face in spite of the daily challenges you all face. From the bottom of our hearts, we thank you and we love you. We realize now that you all are the "face" of the system, the glue that binds it and perhaps the most important people in the day-to-day chain of the patient and family experience. You all face being pulled in a million directions and you all did it with great poise in "high gear." From Ptosha to Laurie and her team at 4-W and some of the ICU nurses like Ben, Alex and Debra, we salute you! We are forever grateful to you all: Michelle, Kari, Genetti, Katie, Amanda, Vicki, Bree, Karen, Janet, Debra, Mary Lee, Janet, Casey, Kacey, Laura, Janice, Jennifer (both of you), Candice, Darius, LaTonya, Allison, Angela, Adrian, Autumn, Simecia, Danielle, Donna, Marty and all of the RN's at Methodist. To the wound care rockstars, Vanessa and Kris; To the RN assistants who were there to help with baths, towels, warm blankets and smiles: Annodgia, LaTasha, Liberty, MaKayla, Carla, Martha and Tamesha--thank you! Also to the excellent ortho techs on the floor: you are wheel chair experts, cord management gurus, "mood elevators", technical wizards--thank you, Leslie, Carl, Roco and Nate.

Finally, to all the caregivers, patients and families out there struggling to find a way through sometimes unimaginable surgeries, illnesses or death... I hope this book has helped you and that you find renewed strength and purpose to fight the good fight with faith and courage. God bless you and may you also find peace, restored wellness and happiness.

# About the Methodist Foundation

_he Methodist Healthcare Foundation is committed to identifying and funding programs that meet the many needs of our patients and their families. We are honored and excited to be part of this project in order to share Amy's tragic-yet uplifting-story in order to help anyone who might need medical care for a family member, friend or even themselves. Together, we look forward to utilizing a portion of the proceeds of this book to help other families who might find themselves in similar situations. It is an important topic that deserves more awareness and we hope to educate and help more in this fight to advocate and promote better medical outcomes for all patients."_

Paula Jacobson, President, Methodist Healthcare Foundation, Memphis, TN

# About the author.

Amy Donaho Howell is the co-author of two other books, "Women in High Gear," and "The Future Belongs to Students in High Gear," both available on Amazon. Amy is the founder and CEO of Howell Marketing Strategies, LLC an established (20 years) marketing and public relations firm in Memphis, TN. Her firm's work includes crisis public relations, marketing and social media strategies for a number of business across industries such as healthcare, banking and finance, real estate, architecture, construction and aviation.

Although she now resides in Tennessee, Amy has also lived in Texas and Alabama and enjoys connecting with diverse people across the social media platform. In 2009, Amy joined Twitter and unlocked the power of key relationships and friendships which include her co-author, Anne Deeter Gallaher of Harrisburg, PA. The story of how they met and collaborated on two books can be found in "Women in High Gear."

Amy is a graduate of Rhodes College in Memphis, TN, where she earned her Bachelor of Arts degree with an emphasis on English and Literature.

She is active in the Memphis community having served on several board of directors as well as being the recipient of civic and fundraising awards. She is passionate about writing, teaching, speaking and has been a keynote speaker at conferences in the Southeast on topics such as social media and best practices for marketing and public relations. She also speaks regularly on both of her "high gear" books. Recently her passion has become patient advocacy and sepsis awareness--a largely undocumented and discussed problem facing our U.S. hospitals.

Amy is married to Jim Howell, and they have two children, Bryan and Abby. The family also includes three dogs and two guinea pigs. When she's not working or writing, Amy can be found somewhere on the Tennessee River. If you want to reach her, you can send a tweet to her @HowellMarketing or @ HealinginHighGear (her Twitter feed dedicated to #Sepsis awareness). Amy's email address is Amy@Howell-Marketing.com.

Complete information can be found on Amy's website at www.howell-marketing.com.

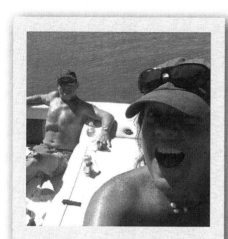

2014, our life before surgery!

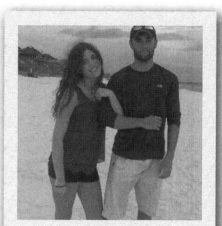

2015, Bryan and Abby:
our rocks

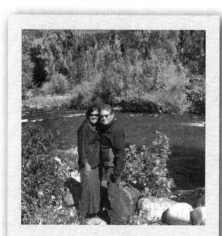

Aspen, 2014 before surgery

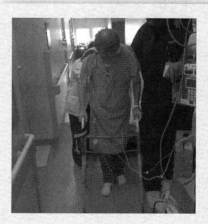

Cord management was often a challenge

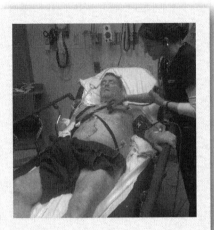

ER fully Septic--when all hell broke
loose: Jan. 25, 2015

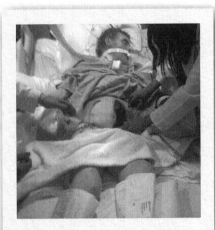

Feb 2015, darkest hours

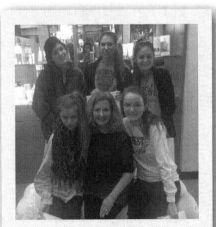

Feb. 8, 2015,
Abby's birthday at Mona Spa

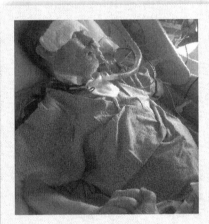

I held Jim's hand often and talked to
him all the time

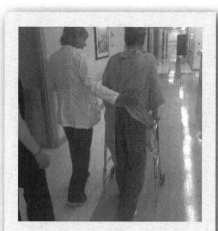

Jim had lots of PT and walking was hard some days!

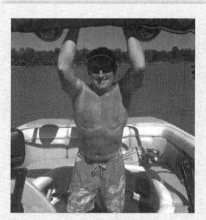

Jim Howell in September of 2014, just months before surgery

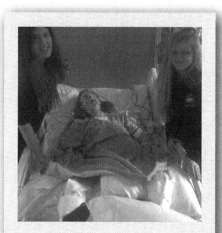

Kids are pillars of strength

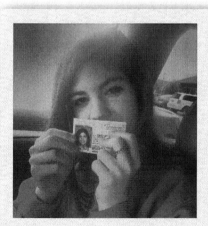

Life goes on...
Abby and her driver's permit, 2015

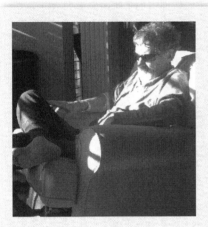

March 4th: the day before
"Hell Day", 2015

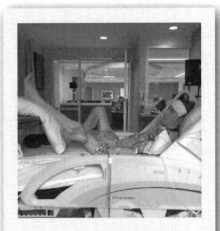

March in ICU—too skinny
for words

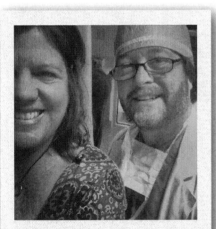

Me and Dr. Miller sharing good news that
Jim made it through surgery

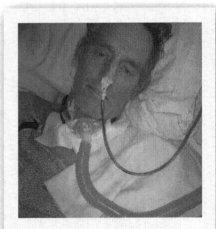

NG Tube be hated!

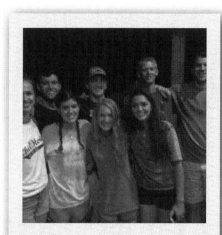

Our fantastic river kids we love

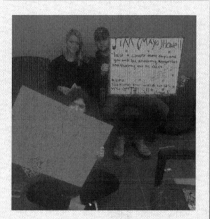

Our kids made posters for
the room

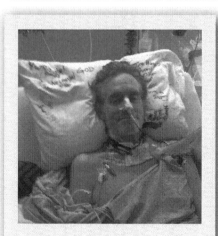

St. Patrick's Day in ICU, 2015

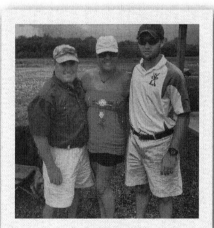

TN State Trap Tourney,
June, 2014 (before surgery)

Made in the USA
Lexington, KY
12 August 2016